Multiple Sclerosis

A Guide for Families
Third Edition

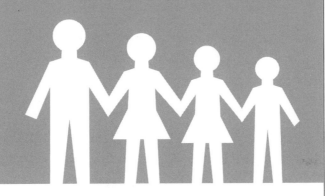

Rosalind C. Kalb, Ph.D.

Demos Medical Publishing
386 Park Avenue South
New York, NY 10016, USA

Designed and produced by Reyman Studio
Copyeditor: Nelda Hills
Indexing: Joann Woy
Printer: Transcontinental

Visit our website at *www.demosmedpub.com*
http://www.demosmedicalpub.com

Library of Congress Cataloging-in-Publication Data

Kalb, Rosalind.
Multiple sclerosis : a guide for families / Rosalind C. Kalb.-- 3rd ed.
p. cm.
Includes index.
ISBN 1-932603-10-7 (pbk. : alk. paper)
1. Multiple sclerosis--Popular works. 2. Multiple
sclerosis--Patients--Family relationships--Popular works. I. Title.
RC377.M842 2005
616.8'34--dc22

2005017657

Printed in Canada

Dedication

To the memory of Labe Scheinberg, MD, a pioneer in the care
of people with MS and their families. He recognized early that
MS affects not only the person who has the disease, but all
those who live with it as well. Dr. Scheinberg devoted his career
to helping people live more comfortably and productively with
MS, and teaching a generation of healthcare professionals the
importance of comprehensive, interdisciplinary care for
everyone affected by this disease.

Contents

Foreword

Why is a guide for families needed?

ALTHOUGH MANY ADVANCES have been made in the understanding and treatment of multiple sclerosis (MS) since 1998,
when the first edition of this book was published, the challenges
for families living with MS continue to be significant. The con-
tributors to the new edition remain committed to providing family members with the information they need to live comfortably
with the disease and with each other.

Multiple sclerosis is typically diagnosed in young adulthood—
the time in life when decisions are being made about marriage,
children, and careers. From diagnosis onward, the disease can
affect the life cycle of the entire family, compounding and confusing the normal transitions and stresses of everyday living. Life
challenges, including marriage, child rearing, job changes, retirement, and the death of elderly parents, are often complicated by
the presence of MS.

What happens when a promising career is detoured, resulting
in the loss of college funds for the children and retirement income
for parents? How does MS affect a person's ability to be the kind
of parent he or she always wanted to be? How do family mem-

bers feel when their roles in the household begin to shift in response to the demands of the illness? How do older couples that are preparing for a long-planned and well-deserved retirement deal with an adult child who returns home with a significant disability? How can a family plan for a future that has been redefined by an unpredictable disease? Multiple Sclerosis: A Guide for Families has been written to address these important questions.

How will this book be helpful for families living with MS?

FAMILIES EXPERIENCING MS often find themselves in uncharted territory. Prior patterns of interacting with one another may undergo major changes. The disease may require shifts in roles and responsibilities that have a significant impact on the lives of all family members. Guilt, anger, sadness, and a sense of burden can become part of the family fabric and create barriers to intimacy, joy, growth, and family unity. This book can help families negotiate their way through these barriers or—even better—find ways to prevent them from developing. This book enables families to move toward a restoration of balance, humor, productivity, and family solidarity. It can lead the way for families, helping them to understand the potential impact of MS on family life, strengthening coping strategies, and planning more effectively for the uncertain tomorrows.

This book helps to provide a feeling of connection for families living with this chronic and unpredictable disease. It acknowledges the confusion and distress that can be experienced by family members and conveys the message that your family is not alone. Hearing this message is an important first step in taking action to get the help and support everyone needs to live comfortably with the challenges of MS. The information in these chapters is communicated by well-known experts in each area. Difficult but crucial topics, including cognitive and emotional changes, sexuality, parent-child relationships, care giving challenges, and the financial and legal aspects of sound life planning, are addressed directly and comprehensively. One goal of the guide is to encourage family members to discuss the disease more openly in order to explore and clarify their individual perspectives on the experience of MS.

The third edition of Multiple Sclerosis: A Guide for Families offers new chapters that address the topics of potential long-term care needs, and the challenges of parenting a child or teen with MS. Other chapters have been expanded and updated to create a dynamic and extremely useful and usable book for families living with MS and the professionals who assist them.

Nancy J. Holland, R.N., Ed.D.

1

When MS Joins the Family

Rosalind Kalb, Ph.D.

T HE VAST MAJORITY of people who have multiple sclerosis (MS) are diagnosed between the ages of 20 and 50 years. The disease thus affects people in their most active years: young adults readying themselves to leave home in pursuit of academic, vocational, or social goals; men and women in the process of launching careers and families of their own; and those in middle age who are enjoying their productive years and planning for their retirements. In each of these age groups, the diagnosis of a chronic and unpredictable disease has significant impact, not only on the individual who receives the diagnosis of MS, but also on the family members and loved ones whose lives are interwoven with that person (see Chapters 6, 8, and 9).

What is it about MS that makes its impact on the family so great?

MS is a chronic disease

ALTHOUGH WE NOW have several treatments designed to modify the course of the disease, we still have no cure for MS. Since the illness has little impact on life expectancy, the person diagnosed with MS will likely be living and coping with its effects for many years. MS has often been compared to the "uninvited guest" who arrives at the door one day, complete with baggage, and never goes home. The guest moves into the household, using up space in every room of the house, and taking part in every family activity.

MS is unpredictable

NO ONE CAN predict with any certainty how a person with MS will fare several years down the road. While it causes severe or incapacitating disability for relatively few, it creates a bewildering question mark for all. Individuals with MS and their family members may have difficulty anticipating what the next day or week will bring, let alone the more distant future. As a result, the established rhythms of daily life can be severely disrupted as family members attempt to respond to the demands of the illness. Planning becomes difficult, creating an ongoing need for flexibility and creativity.

MS is unpredictable not only in the course it follows, but also in the kinds of symptoms it may cause. No two people have MS in exactly the same way. Since the disease can affect almost any system in the body, people feel vulnerable both physically and psychologically. In addition to the more visible symptoms (e.g., walking difficulties or imbalance), MS can cause less obvious symptoms (overwhelming fatigue, bladder and bowel problems, changes in sexual function, visual impairment, and sensory changes), as well as intellectual and emotional changes. "What's next?" is the question commonly asked by individuals and families living with MS. Unfortunately, it is difficult to predict the answer.

MS is expensive

ILLNESS OF ANY kind can be expensive, and a chronic disease that appears during a person's most productive years can have major financial consequences for the entire family. In addition to this more obvious cost in dollars and cents, there is a significant drain on other family resources, including time, energy, and emotions. Families living with MS face the daily challenge of trying to distribute these valuable resources evenly among all family members. MS should not be allowed to sap any more of these resources than it absolutely needs; otherwise, the needs of other family members may go unmet (see Chapter 11).

Emotions

LIVING WITH MS poses an ongoing challenge to the emotional equilibrium of a family (see Chapter 2). Both the person who has MS and family members experience feelings of loss and grief with each new symptom and each change in functional ability. Each progression in the illness requires the entire family to adjust to the loss and redefine themselves accordingly. "Who am I now that I can no longer do some of those things that helped to define me as me?" "Who are we as a couple now that our partnership is being redefined by MS?" "Who are we as a family now that our roles have changed and our relationships to each other and to the community are changing?"

Along with grief comes anxiety over being unable to predict what the future will bring. While all people live with uncertainty, most are not so aware of it on a day-to-day basis. As adults, we tend to take for granted our ability to plan and look forward to events. Families living with MS sometimes feel overwhelmed with "what if's."

Anger can also become a part of life with MS. When uncertainty, change, and loss threaten the family's sense of order and control, individual family members may feel increasing resentment—toward the MS, toward one another as gradual shifts occur in their roles and relationships, and even toward themselves for being unable to do the things they want or need to do.

The ebb and flow of these emotions can take a toll on even the most secure and stable families. Learning to recognize, communicate, and share these feelings with one another helps family members to cope with them more comfortably.

Energy

THE ENERGY DRAIN on families living with MS comes both from the effort required to do things differently and from the emotions that surround these adjustments. Families who have experienced changes in their daily routines because of MS say that "nothing is easy or automatic any more . . . everything takes so much effort." Part of this effort involves finding alternative ways to get things done; part of it involves dealing with the feelings that each person has about having to incorporate these changes into daily life.

Time. MS tends to slow people down. The various physical and psychological symptoms of the disease interfere with the activities not only of the person who has the illness, but also of anyone in the household who shares those activities. Time is a valuable commodity for today's busy families, and the need to slow the pace, postpone activities, or rearrange schedules can produce a new kind of stress for all concerned.

Challenges to Family Coping

FAMILIES EFFORTS TO cope with the intrusion of MS into their lives are challenged not only by the complexities of the disease, but also by the complexities of the families themselves. What is it about families that complicates the coping process?

Individual Needs and Coping Styles

THE FAMILY UNIT is made up of individuals, each with a unique personality and coping style, as well as age-appropriate needs and goals. Each person in the family will see the MS in a slightly different way, and respond to its demands in terms of the way it impacts his or her particular situation. Thus, the MS will mean something different to the husband with MS who can no longer handle his construction job, his wife who needs to take a job outside the home, his young daughter who relies on him to coach the soccer team, and his teenage son who suddenly finds himself with a host of new responsibilities around the house. Therefore, the family's efforts to deal with the disease cannot be seen as a unified, coherent process, but rather as the sum total of individual, sometimes conflicting, coping efforts.

For example, a woman might respond to her diagnosis by wanting to read everything available about MS and its treatments, while her husband and children want to read and think about MS as little as possible. Or, a woman might feel the need to discuss her husband's MS with friends, relatives, and even acquaintances, while he desperately wants to keep it a secret. While each of these coping strategies might be perfectly valid, the difficulty arises from the fact that different members of the family may be trying to utilize them simultaneously.

Similarly, a child's need to know and understand what is happening to Dad may conflict with the family's wish for privacy. Not only do young children have trouble keeping secrets, but they are also unable to appreciate the potential impact of this kind of information on their father's employment or place within the community. As another example, the family's need to engage in effective financial planning may fly in the face of their need to deny the possibility of future disability. In other words, the family's response to the MS is not a simple one. At any given point in time, it is a reflection of the feelings, attitudes, needs, and priorities of each of the people involved.

Disruption Of The Family's Rhythm

OVER THE YEARS, families tend to develop a rhythm of their own—a reasonably smooth and predictable way of carrying out the routines of daily life. Each of the adults in the household has, by spoken or unspoken agreement, taken on certain important functions in the household. As they grow and develop, each of the children also takes on an increasing number of age-appropriate chores and responsibilities. If one person in the family becomes unable to carry out his or her particular role(s), the rhythm of the entire family is upset. Whether it is recognized at the time or not, this shift in roles begins to change the ways in which family members interact and communicate with one another. The disabled person may begin to feel "sidelined"—out of the mainstream of family life. A spouse who needs to take on more and more of the responsibilities in the household may start to feel overburdened and deprived of the old partnership. Young children may gradually find themselves in a caregiver role that threatens their own feelings of security and well-being.

Disruption In Family Communication

TALKING ABOUT THESE kinds of changes within the family can be very difficult for a variety of reasons. First, these changes tend to happen slowly and therefore outside of most people's day-to-day awareness. Families do not talk about them at the time because they are not aware that the changes are occurring. Second, people often have difficulty talking about changes in family life that are caused by symptoms they cannot readily see or understand. A person who is experiencing MS-related cognitive changes or severe fatigue may find it difficult to describe to others how these symptoms are interfering with daily activities. Similarly, family members may become frustrated by their inability to see or understand why family life is not proceeding as smoothly as it once did. Third, family members tend to be quite protective of one another, with the result that painful feelings, questions, and concerns are often left unexpressed. No one wants to open a Pandora's box of stressful issues that have no apparent solutions. And fourth, people sometimes feel that "the less said, the better," as though talking about problems will confirm that they actually exist, and not talking about them will magically make them go away. The result of all this may be the "big, gray elephant" phenomenon. The entire family is tiptoeing around this big gray elephant in its midst and nobody quite knows how to mention it.

Important Resources and the Barriers to Their Use

FORTUNATELY, A VARIETY of resources exist to help families live comfortably and productively with chronic illness (see Chapter 13). Healthcare teams, voluntary health organizations, educational materials, and various types of professional and self-help groups are some of the tools available to support families' coping efforts. Unfortunately, there also seem to be significant barriers to the effective utilization of these resources.

Some of the barriers are social and economic while others are much more personal and emotional. Access to quality healthcare is not universal in this country, and access to professionals with expertise in MS is even more limited. Particularly in this new age of cost containment and managed care, individuals who have MS may feel a growing pressure to monitor and manage their own care (see Chapter 3).

Of even greater concern, however, is the fact that many people do not make use of important resources even when they are readily available. Many families refrain from seeking help because of reluctance to acknowledge the potential impact of MS on their lives, or to think about MS more than is absolutely necessary. They may be afraid that thinking about current or potential problems will somehow make the problems seem more real. Other families seem to feel that seeking outside help or support is an indication of their own weakness or inadequacy; they would rather "go it alone." They do not recognize that these resources are the kinds of tools that might enable them to "go it alone" more effectively.

Recommended Strategies For Family Coping

THE FIRST IMPORTANT strategy of the family should be to give MS, or the "uninvited guest," no more space in the household than it needs. As Dr. Peter Steinglass and his colleagues have so aptly phrased it, "The goal is to find a place for the illness while keeping the illness in its place." A family can develop and thrive only when the emotional and developmental needs of each of its members are being met. The family's balance is threatened when MS is allowed to drain more than its share of the family's financial, emotional, and physical resources. Instead of a family with one disabled member, the result is a disabled family.

Similarly, it is important that the interests and activities of family members not be overly restricted by the disabilities of the person who has MS. In other words, families need to learn how to strike a reasonable balance between the interests and abilities of their disabled and nondisabled members. When guilt feelings cause family members to give up favorite activities in which the person with MS can no longer participate, the entire family may start to feel uncomfortable; the person with MS begins to feel guilty over the limitations on other family members while they, in turn, begin to resent feeling "disabled" by a disease that is not their own. The goal is for families to find a way to accommodate the limitations imposed by MS without allowing those limitations to impact every aspect of family life.

The second recommended coping strategy is often a bit more difficult for families to accept, because it involves hoping for the best while planning for the worst that might occur (see Chapters 10 and 12). Planning for the worst involves learning about the possible ways that MS can affect your life and trying to implement plans or strategies now that would cushion the blow if the worst came to pass. For example, a young woman with MS and her husband are starting to look for their first house. While the most exciting and romantic strategy might be to buy the three-story Victorian they have always wanted, the more practical strategy might be to narrow the choice to houses that are all on one level. Then, in the event that the woman's walking difficulties become more severe, she will be able to enjoy her whole house without feeling restricted to one or another floor. Similarly, a couple in which one of the partners has MS might want to think more conservatively about the amount of money they are putting into savings. The savings will be there as a safety net if the family income is reduced because of disability. If the MS never becomes severe enough to threaten the family's income, the worst that happens is that more money has been put aside for retirement, a child's college education, or a wonderful vacation.

Many families resist this kind of planning strategy because thinking about "the worst" seems too frightening. There is almost a superstition that thinking about these possibilities will make them happen and pushing them out of one's mind will prevent them. Unfortunately, these kinds of beliefs can keep families perpetually off-balance; every exacerbation or change in the person's physical or cognitive abilities feels like an unexpected blow for which family members are totally unprepared. Becoming educated about the potential impact of MS on the family, and taking steps to protect the family's financial, social, and emotional well-being, can help each person feel less vulnerable in the face of this unpredictable disease.

Where Do We Go From Here?

THE GOAL OF this chapter is to provide a general overview of the potential impact of MS on family life. The following chapters explore in greater detail the issues that have been raised here. Each includes descriptions of some of the challenges that can arise as well as realistic strategies for enhancing each family's quality of life—now and in the future.

ADDITIONAL READINGS

National MS Society Publications (available by calling 1-800-FIGHT-MS (1-800-344-4867) or online at http://www.nationalms society.org/library.asp)

Living with MS

Minden Sarah L and Debra Frankel. *Plaintalk: A Booklet About MS for Families*

Someone You Know Has MS: A Book for Families

GENERAL READINGS

Blackstone M. The First Year—*Multiple Sclerosis: An Essential Guide for the Newly Diagnosed*. New York: Marlowe and Co. 2002. www.marlowepub.com

Holland N, Murray TJ, Reingold SC. *Multiple Sclerosis: A Guide for the Newly Diagnosed* (2nd ed.), 2001 [Spanish translation: Esclerosis Multiple: Guia Practica Para el Recien Diagnosticado, 2002]

Kalb R, (ed.) *Multiple Sclerosis: The Questions You Have; The Answers You Need* (3rd ed.). New York: Demos Medical Publishing, 2004.

Kramer D. *Life on Cripple Creek: Essays on Living with Multiple Sclerosis*, 2003.

Pitzele SK. *We are not alone: Learning to live with chronic illness*. New York: Workman Publishing, 1986.

2

Emotional and Cognitive Issues

Nicholas LaRocca, Ph.D.

MULTIPLE SCLEROSIS (MS) affects more than just the ability to walk. It can change the way people feel about themselves and their lives, the way they think, and even their ability to learn and remember. These emotional and cognitive effects of MS are not as visible or as obvious as a cane or a wheelchair. However, the psychological aspects of the disease are no less important than the physical changes that can occur. For many, changes in emotions and/or cognition are the most important problem. This chapter reviews some of the common emotional and cognitive issues faced by people with MS and their families:

- ► *Emotional responses*, including the more common reactions people experience to the diagnosis and to life with MS;
- ► *Emotional changes*, which encompass some of the more complex emotional experiences that are possible in MS; and
- ► *Cognitive changes*, including problems with memory, reasoning, concentration, planning and problem-solving, which can be caused by MS.

The goals of the chapter are to add to your understanding of these emotional and cognitive issues and their impact on family life, as well as to provide some concrete suggestions for under-taking positive change.

Emotional Responses to MS

MS IS A COMPLEX and unpredictable disease. Because no two people are psychologically identical, or experience MS in exactly the same way, each person's reaction to the disease will be unique. Although some of the early research in MS attempted to identify an "MS personality" that would predispose certain individuals to the disease or cause all people who have the disease to act in a certain way, it has been repeatedly demonstrated that no such personality type exists. A person's pre-MS personality, good or bad as it may be, is the same personality he or she will have after MS. And it is with this individual personality, and all its diverse traits, that a person will respond and react to the MS experience.

Some of the prior work in MS also described "stages" that people supposedly go through in their efforts to adjust to the disease. These "stage" models have typically been borrowed from cancer research and do not apply very well to chronic disease. MS is an uninvited and unwanted guest in people's lives that does not go away. As a result, the person with MS does not go through a definite, orderly set of stages culminating in adjustment. Rather, adjustment is an ongoing, lifelong process that ebbs and flows with the unpredictable changes brought about by the disease. Because each individual has a unique style and personal rhythm, which in large part determines how he or she will adjust, it is not particularly surprising that the process of adjustment seems to be more successful and comfortable for some than for others. Let us look at some of the emotional issues that arise as people try to incorporate MS into their lives.

Uncertainty And Anxiety

UNCERTAINTY AND ANXIETY set in as soon as the first symptoms appear. MS can begin in a variety of ways, perhaps with a strange tingling sensation or numbness, sudden loss of vision, or unexplained weakness. Uncertainty surrounds these upsetting and unexplained symptoms. "Is it a brain tumor?" "Am I going crazy?" In some cases, the uncertainty drags on for some time until a diagnosis is finally established. Many people actually experience a brief sense of relief when the diagnosis of MS is confirmed. They are not happy about having the disease, but they are relieved to finally have an answer. In fact, in one study that looked at the diagnostic process in MS, the most anxious and unhappy patients following the diagnostic workup were those for whom no specific diagnosis could be confirmed.

Uncertainty does not evaporate with a confirmed diagnosis, however. Because the disease is unpredictable, people with MS are called upon to adjust to a lifetime of uncertainty about their health. They often do not know how they are going to feel or function tomorrow or next week, let alone several years down the road. In addition, there is uncertainty associated with the disease-modifying therapies that are recommended for relapsing forms of MS. These medications have been shown to reduce the number and severity of attacks and may slow disease progression; they are not, however, designed to reduce symptoms or make people feel better. Because of the way these medications function in the body, it is virtually impossible for any one individual to know the degree to which the disease-modifying medication is "working" at any given time. This much uncertainty can lead to a constant state of anxiety.

The effects of uncertainty and its attendant anxiety can include anger and irritability, indecision, difficulty in planning, feelings of helplessness, and pessimism about the future. Family members inevitably share in these feelings. As a result, all family members may find themselves looking for "anchors"—ways to reduce uncertainty and increase a sense of security and stability within the household.

Adaptation And Adjustment

THE UNCERTAINTY OF the initial symptoms and the brief sense of relief at having a name for them are often followed quickly by shock and disbelief. Deep down, we all think of ourselves as invulnerable to illness. It is difficult for a robust, healthy 30-year-old to accept the fact that he or she has a chronic illness that is progressive and potentially disabling. Most people with MS will assure you that they never really "accept" it (any more than they would accept a lifelong electrical storm that sends periodic lightning bolts into their home). What people eventually seem to do is to confront the reality of the disease and learn to adapt to its presence in their lives. This adaptation is important because without it the processes of coping and effective problem-solving can be short-circuited. Those who struggle to "accept" MS may find themselves mired in frustration as symptoms worsen or new ones are added. This frustration may be heightened by well-meaning relatives and friends who become impatient for the person to "get on with life and stop thinking about MS all the time." Adapting to the presence of MS is an ongoing and challenging process; patience, understanding, and good communication will help ease the process for everyone concerned.

Challenges To The Self-Image

MULTIPLE SCLEROSIS IS a tough pill to swallow, in part because it is so "personal." MS-related limitations can interfere with many cherished abilities, including walking, seeing, controlling the bladder, or driving a car. The person with MS may find many valued facets of his or her self-image undermined by these changes. "If I can't play outside with my kids (go on a class trip . . . coach a team . . . bake a cake), what kind of parent am I?" is the sort of question people may ask themselves. Sadness, frustration, anger, and feelings of worthlessness can ensue. Family members may find it hard to comprehend this intense inner struggle for the survival of a positive sense of self. They may see only its external signs, (e.g., irritability, emotional and social withdrawal), or a loss of interest in everyday activities.

Fortunately, for most people who have MS, disease-related changes *challenge* but do not *overwhelm* the self-image. Why? Because people are usually able to find other parts of themselves that they value, many of which are not physical. A mother with MS, for example, may learn that being a good parent does not just mean cooking elaborate meals or driving car pools, but is more directly related to providing the love and structure that children need to feel secure and realize their potential. A man who prided himself on his athletic abilities may discover a love of reading or a talent for writing that he never knew he had.

Grief

THE PROCESS OF renewing the self-image usually entails a period of grieving for those cherished abilities that have been compromised. Loss is a major issue for people living with MS. Many people feel that they have been robbed of their future. This loss of the future does not refer to premature death, which is rare in MS, but to the loss of their prior expectations for how life was likely to unfold. A person with MS might have had a promising career as a musician or a physician but now must follow a different path.

Grief is a healing and restorative process, but one that is accompanied by pain and sadness. Family members may experience some discomfort during this grieving process since it is often associated with a turning inward and feeling blue. However, grieving is critical to adjustment and may occur many times during the course of MS as the person is called upon to cope with new losses. Moreover, family members will need to do their own grieving, as they experience the impact of MS not only on family relationships and shared activities, but also on their own lives. For some, the grieving process may take a long time and may be accompanied by depression. In fact, it is sometimes very difficult to distinguish a normal grief reaction from clinical depression, which is discussed later in greater detail.

Re-Emergence

DEALING WITH EMOTIONS is an important part of the adjustment and coping process, but it is not the only part. In addition to coping with their emotions, people living with MS are generally called upon to make a variety of concrete changes in their day-to-day routines. When people are first impacted by MS symptoms, the disease may feel like a huge, looming monster that uses all the space in the family's life. There may be so much that needs to be done differently—such as getting from one place to another, managing tasks at home or at work, or enjoying leisure activities—that MS always seems to be in the way and underfoot. As people gradually make the necessary changes, however, and become accustomed to some modified ways of doing things, it becomes somewhat easier to "sweep MS into a corner." Although MS is never going to go away, the family can reach the point where the disease no longer drains quite as much attention and emotional energy. At that point, people are able to continue with their lives, secure in the fact that although MS is a *part* of their lives, it does not have to be the whole of it.

The ability to "sweep MS into a corner"—or "keep it in its place"—may last only as long as the disease is quiet and stable. With each significant change or loss, the disease looms large once again, requiring people to repeat the process of grieving and adaptation. Some have described life with MS as a kind of emotional roller coaster, defined by all the dips and turns of this unpredictable disease.

Stress

THE ISSUES DISCUSSED thus far have one thing in common— they all entail stress. Stress is anything that impinges on us and demands some change on our part that is accompanied by an emotional reaction. Life is full of stresses both large and small, painful and happy. Larger stresses (i.e., losing a loved one, losing a job, or getting married) are often referred to as "stressful life events." The smaller stresses of everyday life, such as getting stuck in traffic or misplacing one's keys, might be thought of as "hassles." Having a chronic disease like MS adds a considerable amount of disease-related stress to the common stresses of modern life. Learning to cope with this increased stress load is a major challenge for individuals with MS and their families.

A major stress that accompanies MS is the fear that stress itself may make the disease worse by precipitating exacerbations. Anecdotes abound concerning sudden and traumatic worsening of MS following major life events. There have been more than two dozen studies that have tried to sort out the relationship between stress and the onset or exacerbation of MS. Some of these studies have found a complex interplay between stress and the immune system, and it has been proposed that stress may worsen MS by promoting the inflammatory process. Sufficient evidence to support such an idea is lacking, however, and the relationship between stress and MS remains far from clear.

Sometimes family members worry that their behavior has somehow caused the stresses that worsened a loved one's MS. Many people with MS have been told to quit working in order to cut down on the stress in their lives, or to simplify their lives in order to avoid stress. *There is no scientific evidence whatsoever to support either of these ideas.* Stress is an unavoidable part of life, and a person can create unnecessary, additional distress simply by trying to avoid the unavoidable. One can, however, learn how to cope with stress more effectively. Better coping is not going to slow down the progression of the disease, but it is likely to make life much happier for everyone.

Solutions

WE HAVE THUS far talked about adaptation and adjustment as if they were natural processes at which we are all skilled. To some extent, it is true that we all have within us the potential to cope with incredible stress and loss. However, there are a variety of ways to realize that potential to its fullest, and no two people (even in the same family) are likely to do it in exactly the same way.

The National Multiple Sclerosis Society offers a wide variety of educational programs and materials for individuals and family members living with MS, as well as a program specifically for the newly diagnosed entitled "Knowledge Is Power" (see Chapter 13 and Appendix A). Although not everyone who is newly diagnosed is ready to become an expert on MS, learning about the illness, both at the time of diagnosis and further down the road, can help restore some sense of control over what is essentially an uncontrollable disease. Focusing on the aspects of the illness that you can control—and acknowledging those you cannot—will enhance your chances of success.

Open communication between family members has been recommended so often that it has become a cliché. However, many forms of family strain can be prevented or relieved by the understanding and sensitivity that come from good communication. Even within the most close-knit families, personalities and coping styles may differ significantly. Thus, two members of the same family may respond to the MS with different, even conflicting, coping styles. Perhaps one wants to avoid all talk about MS and pretend for, as long as possible that it never happened. The other person wants to talk and read about it, go to MS meetings, and meet other families living with the disease. Family members need to acknowledge and respect one another's emotional needs and coping styles. There is no one "correct" way to deal with MS, and adjusting to it may require more time for one person than for another.

Support groups offer many people an opportunity to compare experiences and feel less alone. Family counseling can be extremely helpful, especially if you are finding that achieving effective communication on your own is blocked by angry feelings or different styles of dealing with stress and anxiety. There are many ways to "help nature along" and speed the process of putting MS in its place.

Emotional Changes

THE DISTINCTION BETWEEN emotional *responses* and emotional *changes* is somewhat arbitrary. In the previous section, we talked about some of the emotional responses that are most common in MS (i.e., those that almost everyone goes through at one time or another in the ongoing adjustment process). They are referred to as *responses* because it is assumed that they involve reactions to the altered life circumstances brought on by MS. In this section, some of the less common emotional experiences that can occur in MS are discussed. These include more serious emotional changes, along with a few that have a physiological basis rather than being reactions to the stress of the disease. In reality, there is a great deal of overlap among these various categories of emotional experiences. Moreover, we are often guessing when we attribute a specific cause to any emotion because we do not know for certain what is caused by stress and what is the result of demyelination. You may go through your entire life without experiencing any of the things described in this section. However, if these changes are part of your life with MS, the discussion that follows should help you understand what is happening and why.

Depression

THE TERM DEPRESSION is used in a variety of ways. In everyday language, the term is used loosely to refer to feeling down in the dumps. You might hear someone say, "Oh, she's depressed because she got a C on her final exam." This is not depression in the technical sense, but rather a situational and transient sadness or "dysphoria." In contrast, clinical depression (or major depressive disorder) is a serious and, at times, life-threatening psychiatric condition that meets specific diagnostic criteria. These criteria include profound sadness, loss of interest in everyday activities, changes in appetite and sleep patterns, feelings of worthlessness and/or guilt, lassitude, and thoughts of death or suicide. Major depressive disorder is more common in MS than in either the general population or among other disability groups. Research has shown that upward of half of all people with MS will have a full-blown, major depressive episode during the course of their illness. People are at particular risk for these episodes during exacerbations. The person who is in a major depressive episode may be unable to function and may withdraw from daily life and social interactions.

While such episodes are generally self-limited, there is considerable research showing that medication, either alone or in combination with psychotherapy, can help to shorten the episode and prevent or delay future episodes. In this situation, psychotherapy does not mean going to a support group, peer counselor, or other relatively informal form of intervention. Generally, a psychiatrist should be consulted and psychotherapy may be indicated with a mental health professional (e.g. psychiatrist, psychologist, or social worker).

The antidepressants most commonly used in MS today are the selective serotonin reuptake inhibitors (SSRIs) including fluoxetine (Prozac® and generic formulation), sertraline (Zoloft®), paroxetine (Paxil®), citalopram (Celexa®), and escitalopram HBr (Lexapro®). Other antidepressants used in MS include buproprion HCL (Welbutrin®), venlafaxine (Effexor®), and trazodone (made by several manufacturers), as well as the older tricyclic medications (amitriptyline, desipramine, and nortriptyline, each of which is made by several manufacturers).

Bipolar Disorder

BIPOLAR DISORDER IS a relatively rare condition that is related to depression. It may be characterized by alternating periods of depression and mania, or just mania. Manic episodes are usually characterized by some combination of the following: unrealistic optimism; agitation and/or irritability; hyperactivity; sleeplessness; non-stop or rapid talking; a tendency to start myriad projects that are never completed; and uncontrolled expenditures of money. Bipolar disorder is more common in people who have MS than in the general population. It is generally treated using a mood-stabilizing drug such as lithium or divalproex sodium (Depakote®), although an antidepressant may also be necessary if there are depressive episodes. Manic episodes can be frightening and disruptive for everyone in the family, particularly when uncontrolled spending is part of the pattern. In this situation, legal safeguards should probably be considered to protect the financial stability of the family.

A Word About Suicide

SUICIDE—CONTEMPLATED, ATTEMPTED, and completed—is thought to be more common in MS than in the general population. A study in Denmark found that completed suicide was twice as common among people with MS than in the general public. In recent years, additional interest in this subject has been generated by the controversy over assisted suicide. Thoughts about suicide are so frequent in MS because of the high rates of clinical depression and because of the ways in which MS can erode quality of life and cast a pall over the future.

It is beyond the scope of this chapter to enter into the philosophical debate concerning the "right" to commit suicide. We do know that suicidal feelings may pass when mood improves or one's life situation takes a turn for the better. Thus, the goal for all concerned—those with MS, their family members, and their healthcare providers—should be to ensure that the quality of life is the best that it can be given any limitations imposed by the disease. Effective symptom management and emotional support are essential factors affecting quality of life. All those who live or work with MS need to be aware that active intervention and support are of particular importance at those times when suicide seems like the only viable route.

Mood Swings

FAMILY MEMBERS HAVE long complained that one of the most difficult things to deal with are the mood swings of the person with MS. While everyone in the world probably has mood swings from time to time, people with MS seem to be at greater risk for them. Is this the result of some complex alteration in brain structure, or just the frustration that goes along with disability? We do not know. Whatever the cause, the bursts of irritability, anger, sadness, and frustration can make family life very unpleasant. There is no easy solution to this problem. Family counseling and support groups are often helpful. A mood-stabilizing medication such as divalproex sodium (Depakote®) or one of the SSRI antidepressants is sometimes recommended. Most important are awareness and understanding on the part of all concerned, of the strong feelings that are being expressed. Quite often, exploration of these feelings will suggest possible ways to resolve some of them, thereby improving quality of life for the family as a whole.

Emotional Release

WE HAVE MANY ways to describe the fact that feelings are inherently changeable. In addition to "mood swings," we also refer to *emotional lability, emotional instability,* and even the more pejorative *emotional incontinence.* These terms overlap and are often used to refer to a phenomenon that we will call *emotional release*. Differing from the mood swings previously described, emotional release refers to instances in which a strong emotion seems to "take over" and overwhelm the person in a crescendo of feeling. For example, the person who is thinking or talking about a topic that generates a certain intensity of feeling suddenly becomes choked up and starts to cry. That person is not crying because the feeling of sadness or distress is so intense, but simply because the emotional buildup was strong enough to trigger a crying response that he or she is then unable to control. Although the phenomenon is usually over as quickly as it begins, it can create embarrassment and confusion in a person's professional life, and tension and misunderstandings at home. When emotional release occurs in the context of a family discussion or argument, the strong and sudden release of emotions may precipitate an escalation of the whole situation, leading to raised voices, anger, and alienation.

Although many people take this phenomenon for granted as part of their "personality," it is probably due, at least in part, to demyelination in brain centers that are related to the modulation of emotion. People who experience emotional release have found some simple strategies to be useful. The first step is to become aware of the buildup of feeling and the circumstances that tend to precipitate it. Once the person has developed some skill at this kind of self-monitoring, he or she is often able to catch emotional release in its very early stages, as the feelings are welling up but before they crescendo. At that point, the person attempts to take an emotional time-out, pausing for a few deep breaths, slowing or halting the conversation momentarily, and attempting to prevent the emotional reaction from getting out of hand. At times, we could all probably benefit from this strategy because it may carry the additional benefit of preventing the utterance of statements that are later regretted.

Uncontrollable Laughing And/Or Crying (Pseudobulbar Affect)

EMOTIONAL RELEASE INVOLVES the exaggeration of very real emotion. A different, relatively rare phenomenon involves the experience of episodes of laughing and/or crying that do not seem to be connected to any emotion. A seemingly insignificant or innocuous incident precipitates an uncontrollable bout of hilarious laughter or intense sobbing. The person does not feel happy or sad even though the emotional expression seems to suggest it. It is generally assumed that this phenomenon is a direct result of demyelination in parts of the brain that are responsible for the control of emotions. Because these episodes are so unpredictable and disconnected from actual feelings, the strategies suggested for dealing with emotional release are not likely to be helpful. One group of researchers has found that the antidepressant amitriptyline can be helpful in controlling this unusual phenomenon. Preliminary findings from a large, placebo-controlled trial of Neurodex® (a combination of dextromethorphan and quinidine) in people with MS, indicate that this drug may be a safe and effective alternative. Although no studies have been published, anecdotal reports suggest that the SSRI antidepressants (e.g., fluoxetine (Prozac®) and sertraline (Zoloft®)) may also be useful in treating these episodes. For the family, these episodes can be particularly unnerving. However, by understanding the real nature of this unusual experience, family members may avoid labeling such behavior as "crazy" or deliberately disruptive.

Euphoria

EUPHORIA IS A relatively rare MS phenomenon, in which the person is unrealistically optimistic, happy, and even giggly in the face of seemingly dire circumstances that would make most people profoundly depressed. Euphoria is almost always associated with moderate to severe cognitive dysfunction (discussed in the next section). Because euphoric expression seems to come out of nowhere and tends to be inappropriate to the situation, the euphoric individual is often emotionally "out of sync" with others. As a result, the person may feel emotionally isolated from family members, and they from him or her. Social isolation may make matters worse, and the individual who is severely disabled and euphoric would probably benefit from increased social contact.

Disinhibition And Poor Impulse Control

PERHAPS THE RAREST but most dramatic of the emotional changes seen in MS involves loss of normal behavioral inhibitions and control over impulses. People who experience this problem may be socially or sexually inappropriate, have uncontrollable rages, and may even be assaultive or self-destructive. Such behavior is almost impossible to live with and can lead to criminal charges or involuntary psychiatric hospitalization. For some people, this behavior follows a waxing and waning pattern associated with exacerbations. For others, it is simply part of their day-to-day behavior. There is no evidence to suggest that such behavior is under voluntary control or has anything to do with the person's moral character or values. Instead, it is almost surely a direct result of demyelination in those parts of the brain responsible for inhibition. Disinhibition and poor impulse control may at times be successfully controlled with one of the mood-stabilizing drugs such as divalproex sodium, carbamazepine (Tegretol®), or lithium. However, in extreme cases, hospitalization and/or the use of a major tranquilizer such as haloperidol (Haldol®) may be necessary.

Medication Side Effects

A NUMBER OF MEDICATIONS are used in the management of MS and its symptoms, and many of them can affect mood. These include steroids for exacerbations, baclofen (Lioresal®) for spasticity, pemoline (Cylert®) for fatigue, and the interferon-beta medications (Avonex®, Rebif®, Betaseron®). In the past, little attention has been devoted to the effects of these drugs on mood. Perhaps the most dramatic effects can be seen with steroids. Many people get a "high" while on steroids and actually become manic. In addition, the cessation of steroid treatment often produces transient depression. People who have a history of extreme reactions to steroids, especially if they become "high," may be treated in advance with a mood-stabilizing drug such as divalproex sodium (Depakote®). The depressive reaction at the end of treatment can be treated with an antidepressant, but often it is helped sufficiently by an awareness of its cause and emotional support until it passes on its own.

There has been much discussion in recent years about the possibility that interferon-beta precipitates depression. It is well known that the interferons have the potential to alter mood when they are used in very high doses. However, research concerning the effects of interferon on mood in people who have MS has been inconclusive. Every person reacts differently to drugs. Given the variety of drugs used in MS, and the even greater variety of possible combinations, it is probably wise to be alert to the potential for significant emotional side effects. In MS, there are many forces at work to stir up emotional reactions and changes of all sorts. Careful attention to the potential side effects of treatments can help reduce one source of intrusion into the emotional lives of people with MS.

Cognitive Changes

Multiple sclerosis (MS) is a disease that causes damage to nerve fibers in the brain and spinal cord. Because demyelination occurs in the brains of most people who have MS, cognitive functions can be affected. It is only within the last 20 years or so that MS professionals have acknowledged cognitive impairment as a significant issue for many people with MS and begun to study it intensively. Cognitive dysfunction remains a difficult topic for many people with MS—and their doctors—to think about or discuss. Like the emotional aspects of MS, however, cognitive changes have the potential to affect any and all family issues discussed in this book.

Research has shown that approximately 50% of people with MS have no apparent cognitive changes. Approximately 40% have cognitive changes that can be measured by psychological tests but are only mildly or moderately disruptive of everyday activities (e.g., someone who has to write everything down because of memory problems). A small proportion of people with MS, probably no more than 5–10%, have cognitive changes that are severe enough to seriously disrupt day-to-day life (e.g., a person who cannot manage personal finances because of extreme confusion and disorganized thinking).

What exactly is meant by "cognition?" The word comes from the Latin verb "to think" and refers to the "higher" brain functions such as memory and reasoning, in contrast to more primitive functions such as sensation (e.g., vision, hearing) and motor function (e.g., strength, coordination). In MS, a number of these "higher" functions may be affected. The ones most commonly affected are:

▶ *Memory.* Memory is probably the function that is most frequently cited as being affected by MS. This may be true for a couple of reasons: memory is crucial to almost everything we do; and memory lapses are easy to spot because they involve discrete bits of information and minor disasters (e.g., missed appointments). Memory is a catch-all term that encompasses many processes such as learning information (e.g., studying for an exam) and retrieving information (e.g., taking an exam). In recent years, increasing attention has been focused on "working memory," which refers to the short-term storage of information that is required, for example, to hold a phone number in memory for a few seconds. MS can affect almost any part of the memory process. As a result, people with MS-related memory loss may need to spend more time learning new material if they want to retain and eventually recall it when needed.

▶ *Attention and concentration.* All other cognitive functions depend on good powers of concentration. Attention and/or concentration problems may be manifested as the inability to focus for long periods of time or as extreme distractibility during a task. In MS, it is the more complex forms of attention that seem to be affected (e.g., divided attention tasks, which require a person to pay attention to more than one thing at a time). Because fatigue and stress can also affect these functions, the person with MS may be at very high risk for attention and/or concentration problems.

▶ *Word-finding.* Everyone at some time or other has had trouble thinking of a word or name that was "on the tip of the tongue." In MS, this seemingly innocuous problem can become so frequent that it is very disruptive of normal conversation.

► *Slowed information processing.* People who have MS often say that they are still able to do everything they previously did in the intellectual sphere, but that they have to do it all more slowly. For example, processing more than one "channel" of information at a time may be impossible, particularly if it is all moving quickly. Unfortunately, much of everyday life demands rapid-fire, multi-channel processing with quick shifts from channel to channel. For example, Mom may be sitting in the kitchen balancing the checkbook when the phone rings. Just as she is answering it, the kids start yelling at each other in the next room and someone rings the doorbell. If you add to this scenario a slight slowing of thought processes and response time, and some difficulty walking, you can easily see how an ordinary day in the life of a person with MS can become very stressful.

► *Reasoning, problem solving, judgment.* For some people with MS, the first hint of cognitive loss is not a memory lapse, but a poor judgment call or an inability to perform analytic work that previously seemed straightforward. For example, a securities analyst may find that she is no longer able to juggle all of the factors that need to be considered in developing a stock analysis, or that the time it now takes her to complete each analysis significantly reduces her effectiveness and productivity on the job.

► *Visual-spatial abilities.* Most people freely admit that they have difficulty programming their VCR and assembling those toys labeled "some assembly required." However, MS can seriously impair visual-spatial abilities, including certain functions that are critical to safe driving such as being able to follow directions and quickly process right/left choices.

► *Executive functions.* The ability to organize and execute complex sequences, which is an essential skill for adults, is often impaired in MS. The ability to plan, prioritize, schedule, and implement a complex task (e.g., cooking a Thanksgiving dinner, doing one's income taxes, or completing a project at the office) may thus be compromised, with significant ramifications for both work and family life.

▶ *Other functions.* Because MS can affect any part of the brain, there is no cognitive function that one can safely say is never affected by MS. Some, like language functions, however, do not seem to be as affected in MS as they are following a stroke, for example. While most individuals with MS-related cognitive impairment will experience change in only one or two areas, some people with more severe impairment will experience changes in several different functions.

Impact Of Cognitive Changes

IN AN IMPORTANT study of cognition and employment, it was found that 16% of people with MS-related cognitive impairment were working compared with 44% of an *identical* sample of people with MS who were not cognitively impaired. In other words, cognitive changes are more predictive of a person's ability to remain employed than is physical disability.

Cognitive impairment can have a similarly negative impact on the fulfillment of family roles and responsibilities, especially if memory loss leads to unreliability. Unfortunately, family members are often unaware that MS can cause cognitive problems or they do not connect the changes in behavior they see with the person's MS. Failure to remember things that have been discussed or tasks that were supposed to have been done can cause much family strain. Family members often see these lapses as evidence of an "attitude" problem, insensitivity, lack of concern, or laziness. Teenagers may be quick to recognize and capitalize on a weak memory. ("You told me I could go to that party. Don't you remember anything?") Anger and confusion often accompany cognitive changes because of these misunderstandings and miscommunications. In many instances, the most helpful strategy for the family is to clarify exactly what is going on, and why, and come up with some simple strategies for dealing with the problems brought on by cognitive changes (see page 33).

Research

UNDERSTANDING COGNITIVE DEFICITS is important for family members who are trying to cope with these changes. Much of our understanding has come from scientific research, especially during the last 20 years. What follows is a brief summary of some of that research.

Cognitive changes can affect anyone with MS, whether they have had the disease for 30 years or 30 days and whether they are confined to a wheelchair or running a marathon. In other words, there is little or no relationship between duration of the disease, or severity of physical symptoms, and cognitive changes. Although people who have had MS for a long time, or have a progressive course, are at slightly greater risk for cognitive changes, even those who are recently diagnosed and/or have a relapsing-remitting disease course, can have such deficits. Cognitive deficits can worsen during an exacerbation and lessen as a remission sets in, although the fluctuations in these symptoms appear to be less dramatic than the changes seen in physical symptoms such as walking and vision. Cognitive changes can and do progress like other MS symptoms, but the progression appears to be very slow in most cases. One major study in this area found very little progression over a 3-year period.

Much of the research on cognition in MS has used neuroimaging techniques, especially magnetic resonance imaging (MRI). There is a strong relationship between cognitive changes and the amount of demyelination that has taken place. Some research has also attempted to relate demyelination in specific locations of the brain to particular cognitive deficits. This type of research is challenging because most people with MS have demyelination in a number of locations in the brain. Some interesting findings, however, have begun to emerge.

▶ The right and left halves of the brain are connected by a structure called the corpus callosum. When this structure is extensively demyelinated, people with MS are likely to experience slowed information processing, memory loss, and difficulty with tasks that require the left and right sides of the brain to work together.

▶ When the frontal lobes (areas just behind the forehead that are responsible for thinking and reasoning) are significantly demyelinated, there tend to be problems with memory and executive functions—for example, the ability to organize, sequence, prioritize, initiate, and follow through on a complex sequence of tasks leading to a specific goal.

As research methods become more sophisticated, we will broaden and deepen our understanding of how cognitive function is affected in MS, and work to develop more effective strategies for dealing with these changes.

"Functional" MRI studies have begun to show that during certain cognitive tasks, the brains of people with MS actually behave differently than brains of people without the disease. Areas of the brain that are typically "activated" during certain types of tasks are less activated among individuals with MS. Moreover, areas of the brain that are normally inactive during those same tasks do become activated, almost as if the brain were compensating by shifting gears to get the job done.

Evaluation

THE FIRST STEP in dealing with cognitive changes is to recognize that they have occurred. People with MS often find that others do not take their complaints about cognitive loss seriously. Well-intentioned family and friends will say things like, "Oh, I forget appointments, too. That happens to everybody. . . ." or "We're just getting old!" Such reassurances tend to trivialize and invalidate what is a very real set of problems based on a specific neurologic disease—problems in a different class entirely from those due to human frailty, imperfection, and aging. Unfortunately, physicians often reinforce these denials by the use of very brief "mental status" examinations that fail to detect any but the most extreme cognitive changes. Research has shown that such mental status examinations miss at least 50 percent of the instances of cognitive change in MS.

Adequate assessment of cognitive deficits in MS may require an extensive battery of neuropsychological tests. Such batteries can last from 6 to 8 hours or more and cost upward of $2,000. Briefer screening batteries have been developed, which use a carefully selected set of standardized tests shown to be effective in summarizing the results of the longer batteries. Ideally, the evaluation should be done by a psychologist or neuropsychologist who is experienced in MS, although some speech-language pathologists and occupational therapists perform similar types of evaluations. In addition, it is important to assess other psychological factors such as depression and anxiety that may be contributing to cognitive problems. Such an evaluation should probably be done by a psychiatrist or a neuropsychiatrist, a specialist who has had training in both neurology and psychiatry. A good assessment will let you know where you stand and provide the starting point for planning treatment, career change, vocational rehabilitation, and improved family dialogue.

Treatment of Cognitive Changes

THE IDEA THAT we should try to do something about cognitive changes in MS is almost revolutionary. It is, however, one of the fastest growing areas of MS treatment. Here is a brief survey of some of the options.

Symptomatic Medications

THERE IS AS yet no "memory pill" that can improve cognitive function in MS. A class of drugs called potassium channel blockers (4-aminopyridine (4-AP) and 3, 4 diaminopyridine) have been studied for several years. The potassium channel blockers increase the speed of nerve conduction in demyelinated nerve fibers, leading investigators to think that they might improve neurologic function and cognition. Unfortunately, these drugs can put one at risk for seizures because they speed up nerve conduction. A sustained-release version of 4-AP is currently under study. At this time, however, these drugs are not FDA-approved for general use.

Donepezil hydrochloride (Aricept®) has been approved by the FDA for the treatment of memory disorders in Alzheimer's disease. A recent study of 69 MS patients with memory deficits showed that Aricept® had modest benefits for verbal memory—in this case, the ability to remember a list of words. A larger, multi-center trial of Aricept® has begun, and should provide more definitive evidence concerning the effectiveness of this drug.

Disease Modifying Agents

FIVE DRUGS ARE now approved by the FDA for the treatment of MS—the interferon-beta medications (Avonex®, Betaseron®, and Rebif®), glatiramer acetate (Copaxone®), and mitoxantrone (Novantrone®)—and many more are in clinical trials. Avonex® has demonstrated the most positive benefits on cognition. Results with Betaseron® have been mixed, while the results with Copaxone® were negative. No studies examining the impact of Rebif® on cognitive functions have been reported to date. Although none has shown dramatic benefits for slowing the progression of cognitive dysfunction or reversing its effects, investigators remain optimistic. While many of the earlier clinical trials did not adequately assess cognitive function, recent clinical trials are paying closer attention to cognitive problems. If a treatment is capable of slowing or halting the process of demyelination, it should help preserve cognitive function in people who have MS. The jury is still out on this question, but an educated guess is that the verdict is likely to be positive.

Cognitive Rehabilitation

COGNITIVE REHABILITATION IS a systematic program designed to improve cognitive function; it is conducted individually and/or in groups by a psychologist, speech pathologist, or occupational therapist. Such programs have been common in head injury and stroke for many years, but are just coming into their own in MS. If an MS specialist is not available, a clinician with experience treating mild head injury would be a reasonable alternative since many of the problems are similar.

Compensatory Strategies

COGNITIVE REHABILITATION SESSIONS generally combine exercises and drills to challenge and improve cognitive functions (e.g., memorizing lists of words) with the design and implementation of compensatory strategies for dealing with cognitive changes (e.g., use of a notebook as a memory aid). Like fitness programs, cognitive rehabilitation works best when you have a "personal trainer" to direct and encourage you. However, there are many things you can do on your own to improve your situation.

If your memory is weak, substitute organization. Set up a family calendar and put everyone's activities on it. Buy a loose-leaf organizer (e.g., Day-Runner®, Day-Timer®) and set up sections for appointments, things to do, names, addresses, phone numbers, driving directions, and so forth. Set up a home filing system to keep track of all personal papers. Process incoming mail and other papers quickly to avoid accumulations. Set up checklists for repetitive tasks, such as a packing list for travel or a master grocery list for checking off needed items. Set up a distraction-free "zone" in the house and make sure family members respect it. Establish a fixed storage place for frequently used items like eyeglasses and scissors so you can always find them. Involve the entire family so that everyone assists in the organizational changes.

Conclusion

MULTIPLE SCLEROSIS IS a complex disease with many ramifications for the psychological life of the individual and the family. Adjusting successfully to MS requires understanding and addressing these psychological changes along with the physical ones. There are many resources available for education, evaluation, and treatment. By using these resources to the fullest, the family living with MS can succeed in living more comfortably with an unwelcome but persistent intruder.

ADDITIONAL READINGS

National MS Society Publications
  (available by calling 1-800-FIGHT-MS (1-800-344-4867) or
  online at http://www.nationalmssociety.org/library.asp)
Sanford ME, Petajin JH. Multiple Sclerosis and Your Emotions.
Foley F. Taming Stress in Multiple Sclerosis.
LaRocca NG. Solving Cognitive Problems.
MS and the Mind.

GENERAL READINGS

Kalb R, Miller D. Psychosocial issues. In: Kalb R, (ed.) *Multiple Sclerosis: The Questions You Have; The Answers You Need* (3rd ed.). New York: Demos Medical Publishing, 2004.

LaRocca N. Stress and Emotional Issues. In: Kalb R, (ed.) *Multiple Sclerosis: The Questions You Have; The Answers You Need* (3rd ed.). New York: Demos Medical Publishing, 2004.

LaRocca N, Sorensen P. Cognition. In: Kalb R, (ed.) *Multiple Sclerosis: The Questions You Have; The Answers You Need* (3rd ed.). New York: Demos Medical Publishing, 2004.

3

The Family's Relationship
with the Physician and
the Healthcare Team

Jack Burks, M.D.

M ULTIPLE SCLEROSIS IS a chronic, neurologic disease for which there is not a cure. Until 12 years or so ago, its treatment was limited to symptom management with a variety of medications. Major advances over the past few years are enabling us for the first time to decrease the rate of attacks and slow disease progression. In spite of these advances, however, we still cannot make the disease go away. As a result, the doctor-patient relationship in MS differs significantly from the traditional *diagnosis-treatment-cure* model that often applies to acute illnesses. In a long-term illness like MS, a more comprehensive model, involving *diagnosis + education + collaborative problem solving + support*, begins with a timely diagnosis and continues for the remainder of the person's life (See Table 3.1). This model of care promotes the person's efforts to live comfortably and cope effectively with the ongoing demands of the disease.

In this chapter, the role of the physician in a chronic illness like MS is described, and the model of *comprehensive care* that has gradually evolved in response to the long-range needs of individuals and families living with MS is discussed. Next follows a look at the impact of "managed care" on the comprehensive care of people with MS, and recommendations for ways that individ-

TABLE 3.1

TREATMENT APPROACHES IN ACUTE AND CHRONIC ILLNESS

Acute Illness	Chronic Illness
▶ Medical care involves immediate intervention with predominantly short-term goals.	▶ The goals are generally longer-term.
▶ Physician controls most of the decisions, with little input from the patient.	▶ Healthcare teams educate to promote adaptation, disease management, coping, and stress management skills.
▶ The outcomes are quick and decisive.	▶ Goal setting and decision-making are collaborative efforts between healthcare team, patient, families.
▶ Long-term planning is seldom needed.	▶ Goals are reviewed and revised over time.

uals and families can work with their physician and healthcare team to maximize their own health and well-being.

The Role of the Physician in MS Care

THE EARLY HISTORY of MS care was often characterized by what the late Dr. Labe Scheinberg called the "diagnose and adios" school of medicine. Many physicians, frustrated by their inability to provide patients with a cure, gave them a diagnosis and sent them on their way—to live with MS as best they could. Other doctors were reluctant to give the illness a name, and simply told patients that it was a virus and nothing to worry about or, worse yet, that the symptoms were all emotional and required psychiatric treatment. When physicians shy away from an illness they cannot cure, or withhold vital information from patients and their families, their own discomfort is clearly communicated. The patient and family feel abandoned and burdened with the weight of uncomfortable feelings and unanswered questions.

A meaningful doctor-patient collaboration begins with an accurate diagnosis. Once the diagnosis has been made and explained in a straightforward and understandable way, the person (and his or her family) can begin learning how to adapt to, and cope with, life with the disease. This initial phase of the doctor-patient relationship can, and should, set the stage for the entire therapeutic relationship. Hearing the diagnosis from a physician who conveys the information in a thorough and supportive manner gives the person a greater sense of control and mastery. It conveys the reassuring message that the doctor is there "for the long haul," to help the patient and family members learn to deal most effectively with the disease and manage any symptoms or problems that may arise.

Once the MS diagnosis has been made, the physician's focus shifts to treatment, not only of current symptoms, but also of the disease process itself. The doctor's goal is to help each person live optimally with MS, both now and in the future. Because each patient is unique, the doctor can only achieve this goal if he or she takes the time to understand the person's values, lifestyle and priorities, as well as the current symptoms. Armed with this information, the doctor can begin to educate the person about available treatment options for the short term (e.g., management of specific symptoms) and the long term (e.g., treatment to reduce the number of attacks and slow disease progression). Using a supportive, educational approach, the physician engages the patient and family in the treatment process, working to create an atmosphere that encourages open communication and active collaboration. The respective roles of doctor and patient in this collaborative process are summarized in Table 3.2.

Recognizing that some treatment interventions or medications might be acceptable to one individual but not to another, the physician is prepared to present options while respecting the patient's right and need to be part of the decision-making process. The physician thus conveys to the patient and family the important message that they will not be alone in their efforts to cope with the disease and make meaningful choices for themselves.

TABLE 3.2
PATIENT AND PHYSICIAN ROLES/RESPONSIBILITIES IN MANAGING MS

Patient's Role	Physician's Role
▶ Become knowledgeable about MS and its symptoms.	▶ Be knowledgeable about the diagnosis and management of MS and its symptoms.
▶ Become knowledgeable, proactive, assertive regarding MS care issues.	▶ Seek expert consultation on specific diagnosis or treatment problems if uncertain.
▶ Accept the disease, but only as one aspect of your life; do not neglect other aspects of life.	▶ Provide emotional support to the person with MS and his or her family.
▶ Work to enhance coping and stress management skills to promote comfortable adaptation to change.	▶ Communicate openly and honestly in understandable, non-medical language.
▶ Reassess your priorities and make adjustments as necessary to enhance your quality of life.	▶ Listen well and provide opinions on difficult decisions.
▶ Remain active while realistically assessing employment and other productive activity options.	▶ Support patient's and family members' values and lifestyle decisions.
▶ Commit to a lifestyle that enhances your health, safety, and quality of life (see Chapter 4).	▶ Commit to regular follow-up care (every 3–12 months).

Many people with MS and their family members become overwhelmed at one time or another by the extent of the physical and psychosocial problems that can be created by MS. One of the physician's priorities is to reduce this overwhelming feeling by helping people identify smaller, more manageable problems that have workable solutions. This approach is particularly useful for the family that comes to the doctor demanding, for example, either a cure for the person's MS or that the person be made able to walk again. The family is frightened by the disease and unable to focus on any goal other than total eradication of the problem. Physicians who fall victim to these demands may develop feelings of failure that cause them to withdraw from the family and the patient. Rather than "buying into" the family's demands for a cure or a miracle, the physician must help the family recognize and experience its grief over the losses they are experiencing, and then focus on more specific problems that can be addressed satisfactorily. Careful management of common symptoms (e.g., fatigue, spasticity, pain, bowel and bladder problems, sexual dysfunction, and psychological changes) can significantly enhance a person's comfort, independence, productivity, and overall quality of life.

In this brief description of the doctor's role in the treatment of chronic disease, the family has been mentioned several times. In marked contrast to the doctor-patient relationship in acute illness, which may never involve family members at any point from diagnosis to cure, the ongoing collaborative relationship in chronic illness often involves one or more family members (or "significant others"). Healthcare providers who are experienced in MS care are well aware of the impact of this type of chronic illness on the entire family. From the time of diagnosis onward, patients and family members all need to accommodate the changes brought by MS into their lives.

With careful attention to issues of confidentiality, privacy, and autonomy, the physician, patient, and family members decide who in the family will give and receive medical information, and who will have a say in treatment planning. The rationale for any of these decisions needs to be discussed in detail and *reassessed* as family roles evolve, or whenever changes in the patient's condition or in the family's ability or willingness to participate in the treatment process necessitate a change. Thus, for example, the role of parents in the treatment decisions concerning a 17-year-old child with MS will begin to change as the child grows into maturity and wishes to make more decisions independently. Similarly, family members who were initially less involved in treatment decisions may need to become more involved if the person with MS becomes cognitively impaired to a degree that interferes with the decision-making process.

The "Comprehensive Care" Model in MS

A MORE COMPREHENSIVE approach to treatment grew out of the recognition of the complexity and chronicity of the problems caused by MS, as well as its impact on the entire family. The effects of MS are not only medical, but also social, economic, and emotional. The idea of a solitary medical practitioner working to find a cure or manage all the problems no longer seemed feasible. Rather, the far-reaching impact of the disease required the intervention of a multidisciplinary team, working in a coordinated fashion to help the patient and family cope with the ongoing stresses of MS.

MS centers that provide this type of comprehensive care for patients and their families have emerged in the United States and Canada over the past 30 years. In addition to the physician, this type of team might include a nurse, physical therapist, occupational therapist, speech-language pathologist, psychologist, social worker, recreational therapist, and nutritionist (see Table 3.3). Although the members of the team each tend to focus on different aspects of patient and family care, they share the important goals of education, disease management, and support.

Although individual healthcare practitioners have tended in the past to be *reactive*, responding only to losses and negative events, the role of the healthcare team in MS is a *proactive* one. As soon as the diagnosis is known, the team begins to educate the patient about ways to slow disease progression, manage the symptoms and prevent unnecessary complications. Thus, for example, the person who has MS (and family members) will learn the indica-

TABLE 3.3
THE MS COMPREHENSIVE CARE TREATMENT TEAM[1]

Physician: Diagnosis, treatment, support, referrals

Nurse: Education, training, support, symptom management, coordination of care

---

Physical Therapist: Safety, mobility, comfort, exercise programs, use of adaptive equipment

---

Occupational Therapist: Activities of daily living, arm and hand function, home and workspace modification, cognitive testing and retraining[2]

Psychologist/Counselor: Emotional support, psychotherapy, stress management, cognitive testing, and retraining[2]

Speech/Language Pathologist: Speech, communication, swallowing, cognitive testing, and retraining[2]

Social Worker: Community resource guidance

Vocational Counselor: Career options, retraining

1The "team" may exist within one setting, or be a group of independent professionals who work collaboratively to enhance the health and wellness of the person with MS.

2While using different assessment and retraining tools, each of these pro-professionals addresses MS-related cognitive changes.

tion(s) for a specific treatment, the expected result, and the possible side effects. Realistic expectations for a treatment form the foundation for its success, as well as the success of the doctor-patient relationship.

In addition, the team begins to help the entire family with the coping and adjustment process. During these early months, team members assess the family's existing strengths and resources. The family's ability to cope with the stresses of chronic disease will depend on the internal and external resources they bring to bear on the problem. The healthcare team helps patients and families recognize, appreciate, and utilize all their existing strengths to

---

cope with the challenges that arise. Families also need to learn about resources available in the community. What is helpful for one family may not be helpful for another, but the goal is to provide a menu of options so that families can choose what is most useful for them. The educational process needs to be ongoing in order to meet the changing needs within the family. Information that would have been irrelevant to a family in the early stages of the disease may suddenly take on new meaning as significant medical, economic, or social changes occur.

The family clearly has a central role in this comprehensive model of MS care. The family experiences its own reactions to the diagnosis of MS in one of its members. From the outset, family members are encouraged to express their own sadness and anger over this intrusion into family life. They will be unable to support the patient in any effective way over the course of the illness if they are overwhelmed by their own reactions.

The healthcare team can help families assimilate MS into their lives without allowing personal and family needs to be totally submerged by the disease (see Chapters 1, 6, 7, 8, and 9). Family members are encouraged to pursue personal goals and maintain satisfying outside interests and activities so as not to feel like hostages to MS. Spouses and elderly parents, in particular, can experience guilt over their own good health and their feelings toward the family member who has MS. The healthcare team can lessen this guilt by supporting people's efforts to maintain an independent life beyond the MS. This, in turn, will have reciprocal benefits for the team and the person with MS. Over the course of the illness, family members serve as a valuable extension of the healthcare team. To the extent that they continue to feel good about themselves and satisfied with their own lives, family members can be more effective in their care of the person with MS. This, in turn, helps promote the long-range goal of the healthcare team, which is to promote quality care for individuals with MS, free of unnecessary hospitalizations or treatments, and free of the threat of premature or inappropriate long-term placement.

While the comprehensive, multi-disciplinary team approach to MS care is ideal, it is not always available, especially outside of large cities. Your National MS Society chapter, which can be reached by calling 800-FIGHT-MS (800-344-4867), can refer you to an MS center or to MS-specialist clinicians in your area. The challenge is to find ways to access this multi-disciplinary expertise even if you cannot find it within a single center. There are two primary strategies for accomplishing this:

▶ The first strategy is to locate the MS center that is nearest to you, and consider the possibility of using their expertise on a consultative basis. There are many people with MS who visit a comprehensive center once every year or two for a thorough evaluation and recommendations on treatment. The center then forwards its recommendations back to the person's local physician for implementation. While some physicians might resent the input from the MS center doctors, there are many that find this type of collaboration very helpful, particularly since it may not be possible for them to keep up with all of the latest research and information about available treatments.

▶ The second option is to create your own team of specialists and ask them to communicate with one another about your care. In other words, you make every effort to ensure that your family doctor, neurologist, urologist, physical therapist, and whatever other specialist you might use, know what care you are receiving. Some people accomplish this by asking each practitioner to send reports to the other practitioners; other people maintain a file of their own records, including a complete list of all their medications, and bring them to each doctor's visit. Since the MS nurse is often the person who is most familiar with you and your care needs, she or he may be in an ideal position to help you coordinate your care. The goal of these efforts is to ensure that the various aspects of your medical care are working in some coordinated fashion to help you manage the challenges of MS.

The Implications of Managed Care in MS

How DOES THE comprehensive model of MS care fit with the healthcare reform that is currently happening throughout the

United States? Interactions between doctors and their patients are being re-defined in the face of the growing need for cost containment. *Managed* care is a system for organizing large numbers of healthcare providers within a single corporate structure, with the goal of providing quality services to patients while simultaneously controlling costs.

There are major differences between *traditional* and *managed* healthcare. In traditional healthcare, the patients choose the doctors they want caring for them, and the insurance company pays for all or part of the visit. In managed care, the health organization contracts with healthcare providers to provide services to patients who are enrolled in their insurance plans. The patient must abide by the rules of the plan or face the possibility of not being reimbursed for services provided. Although these rules vary from one insurance plan to the next, they typically require patients to choose from a list of participating providers and use their primary care physician as the "gatekeeper" for access to specialty care. As a result, the primary care physician, rather than the patient or family, decides when consultation with an MS specialist is desirable or necessary. Referrals to specialists are usually for a specific number of visits or a limited time period. In other words, specialists do not provide ongoing care for people in many managed care programs. In addition, services once covered by insurance are gradually being shifted outside the traditional healthcare environment. Thus, although counseling, rehabilitation therapies, and education are still important, the new emphasis is on how to provide care at a lower cost. Financial responsibility for many services is being shifted from the insurers to the healthcare providers, their patients, and the patients' families.

Patients and families with reduced access to MS specialists need an even greater understanding of the issues related to MS and its management, and must work closely with primary care physicians to make certain that their needs are addressed. Primary care physicians who traditionally have not provided neurologic care need to expand their expertise in areas such as MS.

A likely outcome will be that the ongoing or "maintenance" care of a person with MS will be provided in the primary care doctor's office, with referrals being made to specialists for a difficult diagnosis, immunologic therapy, and the management of difficult problems or complications. The patient and family may need to depend more on information from publications, lectures, the Internet, voluntary health organizations (e.g., National MS Society, the Multiple Sclerosis Association of America, United Spinal Association), and other resources, to make certain that they are aware of the latest developments in MS. Prepared with this information, it is appropriate (even important) for a patient or family member to ask the primary care physician for a referral to a specialist when they perceive that he or she is unfamiliar with available treatment strategies or is unwilling to pursue additional treatment options.

Is managed care good or bad? Medical treatment managed in this way may initially reduce overall healthcare costs. It is yet to be determined whether it will reduce costs in the long run, or how it will affect the quality of MS-related care. Although managed care seems to provide adequate and cost-effective preventive medicine and treatment for acute illnesses, managed care has yet to demonstrate its effectiveness in chronic diseases, including MS. Specialists in MS care have concerns about the quality of care given to MS patients by healthcare providers who lack experience and expertise in the management of disease symptoms and who may not understand the potential complications of the disease or the side effects of various medications.

The new immunosuppressive treatments in MS have provided an interesting point of contrast between managed care and MS care provided in comprehensive specialty centers. Once patients with MS have been started on disease-modifying medications such as Betaseron®, Avonex®, Copaxone®, or Rebif®, their ongoing care is typically provided by physicians who are not MS specialists. These physicians are often less familiar with the subtleties of treatment, patients' emotional reactions to medications or the injection process, and the management of side effects. Not too surprisingly, one study demonstrated that the dropout rate for one of the medications was much lower for patients who are followed by MS specialist physicians and nurses than for those patients who were being followed by other healthcare providers. This clearly has significant implications for the health and well being of people with MS. The effectiveness of the new immuno-suppressive therapies will ultimately be determined by the ability of patients to use and tolerate them over a long period of time. Simply prescribing a treatment is not enough; teaching patients how to use it and supporting their efforts to continue doing so are essential.

In the long run, the effectiveness of managed care for people with MS will depend on the degree to which patients and families believe that they have access to the kind of treatment and support they need in order to manage their symptoms and live comfortably with MS. A close working relationship between primary care doctors and MS specialists has proved quite successful in the past. The question will be whether this kind of collaboration can continue to flourish under managed care.

An alternative to the comprehensive model in MS care, known as "principal care," is currently gaining momentum. In this model, the MS specialist provides ongoing care, while referring the patient to the primary care physician for non-MS medical care. Some managed care insurance plans are becoming more amenable to specialists providing the comprehensive care.

Whichever approach takes hold in the days ahead, it will be important for individuals who have MS or other chronic illnesses to make their needs and feelings known to their insurance companies. Since people live to an older age and survive for longer and longer periods with diseases like cancer and AIDS, chronic illness is becoming much more prevalent. In order for insurance companies to be able to survive, they must meet their clients' needs and become responsive to this growing segment of the population. Although the pendulum of healthcare management and insurance reimbursement is unlikely to swing back very rapidly, it will eventually respond to the demands of educated and assertive consumers. Consumers will be the ones who educate insurance companies about the unique and ongoing needs associated with chronic illness.

Taking Responsibility for Optimizing Your Medical Care

Choosing Your Physician And Healthcare Team

WHETHER OR NOT your choice of physician is restricted by your health plan, the most important factors in your selection should be (1) your comfort level in working and communicating with this doctor, and (2) the physician's knowledge and experience in MS. Centers that specialize in MS care are often in a position to offer a wider range of medical and psychosocial interventions. However, even the most sophisticated MS center will not meet your needs if you do not feel able to communicate and work comfortably with the healthcare team.

If your healthcare plan requires you to select a primary care physician (most likely an internist, or a general or family practitioner) to act as gatekeeper for your medical care, look for a physician who currently treats other MS patients and is familiar with the complexities of the disease. He or she should be willing and able to help you manage your symptoms and knowledgeable about existing treatment options. The primary care physician should also be willing and able to refer you to a specialist when the need arises. If you are unable to find a physician within your network who is experienced in the care of MS patients, your next best option may be to find one who is willing to learn.

Staying Informed

PEOPLE WITH MS and their family members need to educate themselves about the disease and existing treatment options. In particular, those patients whose care is provided by non-MS specialists need to take responsibility for staying informed and up-to-date about MS management. This is the most effective way to ensure that you are receiving optimal care. Today, more than ever, there are numerous avenues for obtaining this kind of information, including books, newsletters, information lines sponsored by pharmaceutical companies, the Internet, and the vast array of publications offered by the MS societies. Keep in mind, however,

TABLE 3.4
TIPS FOR MAKING THE MOST OF DOCTOR VISITS

▶ Make a list of questions and concerns before the visit.

▶ Prioritize the list and discuss your most important issues first.

▶ Make sure that your doctor has a complete list of all the medications you are taking, including any that have been prescribed by another physician for non-MS-related conditions, and *any over-the-counter drugs or supplements.*

▶ Bring up all your concerns—even the ones that may be difficult to talk about (e.g., bladder and bowel problems, sexual changes, cognitive changes).

▶ Discuss any medication side effects you are experiencing.

▶ Ask for a referral if you would like a second opinion on any aspect of your disease or its management.

▶ Consider bringing a family member or friend to your visit if you feel the need for a "second pair of ears"; consider tape recording the visit for later review.

▶ Ask for more time or another appointment if you have not addressed your issues fully.

---

that some sources are more authoritative than others, and that you cannot believe everything you hear. This educational process will enable you to be an active and informed participant in your own care. The Additional Readings and Recommended Resources sections in this book are an excellent place to start.

Use Your Visits to the Doctor Effectively

THE DOCTOR-PATIENT collaboration is at its most active during the office visit. This is the time to give your physician the information he or she needs in order to help you manage your

TABLE 3.5
CONSIDERING THE IMMUNE-MODULATING THERAPIES

▶ Because MS is likely to progress without treatment, and irreparable damage can occur even early in the disease course, treatment should be considered for any person with relapsing MS even if a person is relatively symptom-free and "feeling fine."

▶ Early treatment improves a person's chances of reducing the attack rate and slowing disease progression over the long-term.

▶ All of the approved treatments are beneficial; the evidence indicates that some may be stronger than others; together, your physician and you can determine the best treatment option for you.

▶ While every treatment may have side effects, 90% of people can learn how to manage the treatments comfortably. If you are having difficulty with your immune-modulating medication (or any other that has been prescribed for you), do not stop taking it without talking to your physician; most problems with treatment can be successfully resolved.

MS. Be prepared for your visits (see Table 3.4 for a summary of recommendations).

Because most people find it difficult to remember all the things they want to talk about, particularly when they are trying to listen to what the doctor is saying, it is a good idea to bring a list of topics and questions. Let the doctor know how current medications are working for you and what, if any, problems or side effects you are having with them. This is particularly true in relation to the approved immune-modulating therapies—the interferons (Avonex®, Betaseron®, and Rebif®), glatiramer acetate (Copaxone®), and mitoxantrone (Novantrone®). Table 3.5 outlines the current thinking among many MS specialist physicians and the National MS Society concerning the use of these therapies (see also the National MS Society's Disease Management Consensus Statement—available online at http://www.national mssociety.org/Sourcebook-Early.asp or by calling 1-800-FIGHT-MS). An effective collaboration between you and your healthcare team will help to ensure that you initiate treatment at the time that you and they feel is most appropriate, and that you can continue comfortably with the treatment for the foreseeable future.

Describe your symptoms, taking care to let the doctor know which of them are causing you the greatest difficulty. Patients are sometimes hesitant to bring up certain issues that they find embarrassing. Unfortunately, some physicians may be reluctant to bring up the very same topics. People living with MS need to know that bladder and bowel symptoms, sexual difficulties, and cognitive and emotional changes can all be significant problems related to their disease. Do not hesitate to talk about them, and do not hesitate to think about looking for another physician if you feel that you are not getting adequate help with these important problems.

Many people with MS use various types of *alternative* treatments in an effort to manage their symptoms—sometimes *instead* of mainstream medicine, but more commonly as an adjunct to the treatments prescribed by their physicians. Alternative therapies include a broad range of treatments (i.e., dietary supplements, homeopathy, chiropractic, and many others). It is extremely important that you let your physician know about any treatments you are using, including over-the-counter medications and nutritional supplements, so that he or she can alert you to potential drug interactions or other risk factors.

Bringing a family member or friend to your doctor's visits can often be quite helpful. People sometimes feel anxious while talking to the doctor and find that they have difficulty focusing on what is said, and even more difficulty remembering it afterward. You might ask your relative or friend to jot down notes for you during the appointment so that you can go over them again later. This person might also be able to remind you of problems or symptoms that have slipped your mind. A family member may have questions of his or her own pertaining to your symptoms or to family issues relating to the illness. In addition to, or instead of, bringing someone with you to the appointment, you might want to tape record the conversation for later review or to share with family members.

You may hear or read about a treatment that seems relevant to your MS or to a particular symptom you are having. It is appropriate to ask your doctor whether this treatment might be helpful for you. If your doctor is not familiar with the particular treatment, it is reasonable for you to ask that he or she look into it further and give you an opinion about it. Doctors who are not MS specialists should be willing to investigate possible MS treatments or make a referral to a specialist who might be more familiar with them.

No matter which topics are covered in a particular visit to the doctor, you should leave feeling that you have conveyed and received whatever information is needed for you to continue managing your MS symptoms and day-to-day activities as comfortably and effectively as possible. If, at the end of your visits, you wonder what has been accomplished, it is time to think about what needs to change in order for those visits to be more productive. If every visit to the doctor is a search for "the cure," the visit is not likely to be a fruitful one. If, however, you are working with your doctor to keep your life comfortable, active, and productive, you have a much higher likelihood of success.

ADDITIONAL READINGS

National MS Society Publications
> (available by calling 1-800-FIGHT-MS (1-800-344-4867) or
> online at http://www.nationalmssociety.org/library.asp)

Early Intervention. Disease Management Consensus Statement.
Foster V. Choosing the Right Health-Care Provider.
Clear Thinking about Alternative Therapies.
Nowack DM. Food for Thought: MS and Nutrition.
Bowling A, Stewart T. Vitamins, Minerals, and Herbs in MS: An
> Introduction.

GENERAL READINGS

Bowling A. *Alternative Medicine and Multiple Sclerosis.* New York: Demos
> Medical Publishing, 2001.

4

Sexuality and Intimacy in Multiple Sclerosis

Frederick Foley, Ph.D.

S EXUALITY IS AN integral part of each of us. It is biologically woven throughout our cells, tissues, and organs, influencing the development and function of the brain and immune system. Sexuality impacts our identity and personality, the nature of our interpersonal relationships, and our life span. Sexuality is depicted in the language, art, laws, music, religion, literature, and culture of every human society. It is omnipresent and universal, yet we each experience it in very different ways. Our individualized experience of sexuality is a continuous process of change and development from birth to death. The presence of a physical illness such as multiple sclerosis (MS) has the potential to complicate the lifelong course of sexual development and the ways in which one defines and expresses one's sexuality.

Many of the early studies on the nature and frequency of sexual problems in MS were of questionable quality. In general, they included too few people to provide meaningful results, used groups that were not representative of the MS population as a whole, and did not involve comparisons with a non-MS control group. In addition, many of the early studies used poorly constructed surveys to gather the information, and tended to focus almost exclusively on men with MS.

In 1999, Zorzon and his colleagues published the first case-control study of MS-related sexual dysfunction. In a comparison of 108 men and women with definite MS, 97 with other chronic diseases, and 110 healthy individuals, the investigators found that 73% of the people with MS reported some type of sexual dysfunction, as compared to 39% of those with other chronic diseases, and 13% of the healthy control group. Among the participants with MS, more men than women reported changes in sexual function.

The Nature and Frequency of Sexual Dysfunction in Women

IT IS IMPORTANT to look at MS-related sexual problems within the context of society as a whole. Studies of the frequency of sexual complaints among women in the general U.S. population indicate that as many as 43% have problems that cause at least "occasional" concern. The few epidemiologic studies on sexual dysfunction in women with MS have reported a wide range of sexual concerns that seem to occur with varying frequencies. At least 50% of women in each of these studies reported problems or changes in their sexual functioning. The most common complaints were fatigue, a decrease in sexual desire, genital sensation and vaginal lubrication, and loss of orgasm. In several studies, a correlation was found between sexual difficulties and overall level of disability. In several of the most recent, methodologically-sound surveys, approximately 80% of women with MS reported at least one sexual problem, although over half of the women surveyed reported little concern about their sexual difficulties.

The Nature and Frequency of Sexual Dysfunction in Men

IN SURVEYS OF the general U.S. population, between 5 and 30% of men under 40 report sexual problems. Studies of men over 40 have yielded more frequent complaints, with 15-52% reporting sexual problems. Chronic disease, as well as alcohol, illegal drugs, and nicotine use, are factors that are associated with an increased risk of sexual problems.

As with women, surveys on the prevalence of sexual dysfunction in men with MS vary widely in their findings. Difficulty acquiring or maintaining satisfactory erections seems to be the most common male complaint in MS, with frequencies ranging from 25-80% of those surveyed. These observations are noteworthy in comparison to a 5% occurrence rate of erectile dysfunction in healthy 40-year-old men in the general population, and a 15-25% occurrence rate after age 65. The combined findings of numerous studies on the causes of erectile dysfunction in MS suggest both a physical and a psychogenic (emotional) role in MS-related erectile dysfunction.

In addition to erectile problems, surveys of men with MS have identified decreased genital sensation, fatigue, difficulties with ejaculation, and decreased interest or arousal as fairly common complaints. In the study by Zorzon and his colleagues, one of the most comprehensive and methodologically sound surveys to date, only 35% of men reported no sexual problems, and many reported multiple problems. This study also found that the majority of men who experienced sexual problems believed that these problems had a noticeable impact on their intimate relationship.

Primary, Secondary, and Tertiary Sexual Dysfunction

THE WAYS IN which MS can affect sexuality and expressions of intimacy have been divided into *primary*, *secondary*, and *tertiary* sexual dysfunction. Primary sexual dysfunction is a direct result of neurologic changes that affect the sexual response. In both men and women, this can include a decrease in, or loss of, sex drive, decreased or unpleasant genital sensations, and diminished capacity for orgasm. Men may experience difficulty achieving or maintaining an erection, and a decrease in, or loss of, ejaculatory force or frequency. Women may experience decreased or absent vaginal lubrication.

Secondary sexual dysfunction stems from nonsexual MS symptoms that can also affect the sexual response (e.g., bladder and bowel problems, fatigue, spasticity, muscle weakness, body or hand tremors, impairments in attention and concentration, and nongenital sensory changes).

Tertiary sexual dysfunction is the result of disability-related psychosocial and cultural issues that can interfere with one's sexual feelings and experiences. For example, some people find it difficult to reconcile the idea of being disabled with the idea of being fully sexually expressive. Changes in self-esteem and self-perceived body image, demoralization, depression, or mood swings can all interfere with intimacy and sexuality. Partnership changes within a relationship (i.e., one person becoming the other's caregiver) can severely challenge the sexual relationship. Similarly, changes in employment status or role performance within the household are often associated with emotional adjustments that can temporarily interfere with sexual expression. The strain of coping with MS challenges most partners' efforts to communicate openly about their respective experiences and their changing needs for sexual expression and fulfillment.

Primary Sexual Dysfunction (Resulting From Neurologic Impairment)

⊙ Evaluation and treatment

COPING WITH PRIMARY sexual dysfunction can be facilitated by discussing symptoms with a health professional who is knowledgeable about MS. The first step in any kind of treatment is a thorough evaluation to diagnose the difficulty. The evaluation process may include: a physical history and examination; a review of current MS and other medications for their possible effects on sexual functioning; a detailed sexual history; and perhaps some specialized tests of sexual function. The sexual history thoroughly examines the current problem and investigates both present and prior sexual relationships and behaviors. The specialist may wish to conduct a joint interview of the person who has MS and his or her sex partner in order to gain a better understanding of the problem as it is experienced by both individuals. A number of questions may be asked regarding the couple's communication, intimacy, and sensual or erotic behaviors in order to obtain a balanced view of their relationship. When this has been accomplished, treatment may begin with feedback from the assessment process, education about the effects of physical symptoms of MS, and suggestions for managing these symptoms.

⊙ Decreased vaginal lubrication

SIMILAR TO THE erectile response in men, vaginal lubrication is controlled by multiple pathways in the brain and spinal cord. Psychogenic lubrication originates in the brain and occurs through fantasy or exposure to sexually-related stimuli. Reflexogenic lubrication occurs through direct stimulation of the genitals via a reflex response in the sacral (lower) part of the spinal cord. Psychogenic lubrication can be enhanced by establishing a relaxing, romantic, and/or sexually stimulating setting for sexual activity, incorporating relaxing massage into foreplay activities, and prolonging foreplay. Reflexogenic lubrication can sometimes be increased by manually or orally stimulating the genitals. Decreased vaginal lubrication can be dealt with easily by using generous amounts of water-soluble lubricants, such as K-Y Jelly®, Replens®, or Astroglide®. Health care professionals do not advise the use of petroleum-based jellies (e.g., Vaseline®) for vaginal lubrication, because they greatly increase the risk of bacterial infection.

Because women have erectile tissue in the clitoris, which functions similarly to the male erectile tissue, sildenafil (Viagra®—see description under erectile function) has been studied in women, including those with MS, to see if this medication would help with lubrication and other aspects of the sexual response. The results of all trials with women, however, have been negative. Having concluded that the female response is more complex and multi-determined than the male response, the manufacturers of Viagra® recently terminated all trials in women.

⊙ Sensory changes

UNCOMFORTABLE GENITAL SENSORY disturbances, including burning, pain, or tingling, can sometimes be relieved with prescription medications such as carbamazepine (Tegretol®) or phenytoin (Dilantin®). The application of a cold compress prior to sexual activity can sometimes suppress uncomfortable sensations. Decreased vaginal and clitoral sensation can sometimes be overcome by more vigorous stimulation, either manually, orally, or with the use of a vibrator. Strap-on clitoral vibrators may be worn by the woman or attached to the base of the penis during intercourse, allowing for more intense clitoral stimulation. In general, AC electric plug-in vibrators have more powerful motors and are more stimulating than DC-powered battery-operated ones. However, some electric vibrators are quite powerful and can irritate vaginal or clitoral tissue if they are applied too vigorously. (A large selection of vibrators and other sexual aids have become more readily available in recent years due to the proliferation of mail-order services that allow people to shop conveniently and privately at home. Some mail-order companies are sensitive to the needs of people with physical disabilities and can be good sources of information for selecting sexual aids. See the Recommended Resources at the end of the chapter.) Exploring alternative sexual touches, positions, and behaviors, while searching for those that are the most pleasurable, is often very helpful. Masturbation with a partner observing or participating can provide important information about ways to enhance sexual interactions.

⊙ Problems with orgasm

MS CAN INTERFERE directly or indirectly with orgasm. Primary orgasmic dysfunction stems from MS lesions in the spinal cord or brain that directly interfere with orgasm. In women and men, orgasm depends on nervous system pathways originating in the brain (the center of emotion and fantasy during masturbation or intercourse), and pathways in the upper, middle, and lower parts of the spinal cord (which control sensations from erogenous zones such as lips, nipples, penis or clitoris, and so forth). If these pathways are disrupted by plaques, sensation and orgasmic response can be diminished or absent. In addition, orgasm can be inhibited by secondary (indirect) symptoms, such as sensory changes, spasticity, cognitive problems, and other MS symptoms. Tertiary (psychosocial or cultural) orgasmic dysfunction stems from anxiety, depression, and loss of sexual self-confidence or sexual self-esteem, each of which can inhibit orgasm.

Treatment of orgasmic loss in MS depends on understanding the factors that are contributing to the loss. If sensation is disturbed in the genitals and lower body areas, increasing stimulation to other erogenous zones, such as breasts, ears, and lips, may enhance the orgasmic response. Conducting a sensory "body map" with one's partner, to explore the exact locations of pleasant, decreased, or altered sensations, can be both intimate and informative (see body mapping exercise on pp. __–__) Sometimes stimulating the edges of body zones that are experiencing numbness or diminished sensation can feel sensually or erotically pleasing. Similarly, increasing cerebral stimulation by watching sexually-oriented videos, exploring fantasies, and introducing new kinds of sexual play into sexual activities can help trigger orgasms.

⊙ Decreased libido

ONE OF THE most difficult primary sexual symptoms to compensate for is loss of sexual desire (libido), which is one of the most common sexual changes among women with MS. When loss of desire is due to secondary sexual dysfunction (e.g., as a result of fatigue) or tertiary sexual dysfunction (e.g., as a result of depression), treatment of the interfering secondary or tertiary symptoms frequently restores libido. When a person's libido is diminished by MS, he or she may begin to avoid situations that were formerly associated with sex and intimacy. Sexual avoidance serves as a source of misunderstanding and emotional distress within a relationship. The partner may feel rejected, and the person with MS may experience anxiety, guilt, and reduced self-esteem. Misunderstandings surrounding sexual avoidance frequently compound the loss of desire and diminish emotional intimacy in relationships.

Restoring libido in the context of an intimate relationship

begins by focusing on the "sensual" and the "special person" aspects of the relationship. Sensual aspects include all physically and emotionally pleasing, non-erotic contact, such as backrubs, handholding, and gentle stroking of the face, arms, and other nongenital body zones. During periods of diminished sexual drive, sex partners often neglect these sensual, non-sexual aspects of their physical relationship. Making a date for a non-sexual but sensual evening can enable partners to enjoy each other physically and engage in enjoyable sensual exploration of each other's bodies without the pressure of working toward sexual intercourse. In essence, sexuality has to be "relearned" when the central nervous system has compromised libido. Relearning one's sensual nature is a critical first step in the process.

The special person aspects of a relationship include all those behaviors that one engages in to show the other person that he or she is special and important. Loving gestures from an earlier, "romantic" phase of a relationship, such as unexpected flowers, a surprise note in a lunch bag, or a spontaneous, affectionate hug, tend to be forgotten amidst the pressures of raising children, developing careers, and coping with MS symptoms and disabilities. Restoring or increasing these special acts toward one another can help set the stage for increasing intimacy which can, in turn, sometimes stimulate new libido.

For the person without a current sexual partner, exploring one's sensual and erotic body zones is an important step in restoring libido. Combining enjoyable cerebral sexual stimulation (achieved via fantasy, sexually explicit videos, books, and so forth) with masturbation or sensual, physical self-exploration is sometimes helpful. Using a vibrator or other sexual toys may complement these efforts. Although beginning to work on restoring libido may feel like an unrewarding "chore" when there is no intrinsic sex drive, working toward rekindling this vital aspect of "self" can be an important aspect of coping with MS.

Kegel exercises are sometimes prescribed to enhance female sexual responsiveness (although these exercises have not been tested in a clinical trial to determine whether they are helpful in MS). To perform the Kegel exercise, the woman alternately tightens and releases the pubococcygeus muscle (identifiable as the muscle that starts and stops the urine flow in midstream). Exercising this muscle several times a day is recommended in an effort to enhance muscle tone and responsiveness. The rationale for Kegel exercises is that sensation from the muscles around the vagina is an important part of erotic sensation, and female orgasm consists of contractions in several of these muscles.

Currently there are no medicines available to treat loss of libido in women with MS, although there are several medicines in pre-clinical and phase I clinical trials that are being tested to see if they will enhance libido in women without MS. These medicines work by stimulating different pathways and structures in the brain that seem to be related to sexual drive and desire. However, it will take a number of years before it is known whether they are safe and effective.

Some men and women who have sustained loss of libido report that they continue to experience sexual enjoyment and orgasm even in the absence of sexual desire. They may initiate sexual activities without feeling sexually aroused, knowing that they will begin to experience sexual pleasure with sufficient emotional and physical stimulation. This adaptation requires developing new internal and external "signals" associated with *wanting* to participate in sexual activity. In other words, instead of experiencing *libido* or *physical desire* as an internal "signal" to initiate sexual behaviors, one can experience the anticipation of closeness or pleasure as an internal cue that may *lead to* initiating sexual behaviors and the subsequent enjoyment of sexual activity.

BODY MAPPING EXERCISE

The following steps explain the exercise:

1. Conduct the exercise (initially by oneself) lying down naked in a comfortable, safe, distraction-free setting (e.g., bedroom). Begin by gently touching the top of the head with the fingertips, noticing the sensations. Systematically move down the face and head, and then the body, slowly touching as much of oneself as is comfortable. Take notice of all sensations, and vary the pace and pressure of the movements with the goal of learning what feels pleasurable and what does not. Do not be

overly concerned about feeling sexual, and do not attempt to reach orgasm. The purpose is to explore yourself and to develop an enhanced sensual awareness of pleasurable touch. Many people may initially experience sadness or irritability when they conduct the exercise, as they process the sense of emotional loss associated with libido changes, particularly when they stroke their genitals. Some find it helpful to conduct the exercise in front of a mirror in order to provide additional visual feedback. Conduct the exercise for 15 to 20 minutes approximately twice a week.

2. Include the partner after the first few sessions of self-exploration. When libido diminishes or is absent, the sequence of communications around sexual behaviors for partners almost always needs to change as well. Conducting the body mapping exercise for the purpose of *improving communication* (rather than for immediate sexual gratification) allows the partners to develop new sequences of touch that are mutually pleasing. It also allows for communicating about the emotions associated with this process. Partners should be instructed verbally (e.g., "stroke me lightly on my neck with just your fingertips") and nonverbally (e.g., taking the partner's hand and guiding it to a pleasurable place, demonstrating the pace and pressure of the desirable touch). For the first two or three times the partner is included, touching the genitals should be avoided.

3. Expand the body mapping exercise with the partner to include stimulating the genitals. The focus should remain on communication and the restoration of pleasure, without the goal of having intercourse or achieving orgasm.

4. If he or she is physically able, the person with MS should reciprocate by conducting a body mapping exercise on the partner. This introduces mutual communication and sensual pleasure during the process of relearning cues associated with sexual pleasure. Partners can take turns, spending 15 to 20 minutes each, as "givers" and then "receivers" of pleasure. In the role of receiver, the goal is to suspend the usual concern for the partner's pleasure and focus on communicating to the partner how he or she can provide maximal pleasure. Similarly,

in the role of giver, the goal is to be maximally attentive and completely devoted to following the cues and feedback offered by the partner. Changing one's sexual signals or cues to initiate sexual activity can be assisted by conducting a body mapping exercise. Body mapping is typically used to help compensate for primary (genital) or secondary (nongenital) sensory changes, but it can be a useful first step in the enhancement of physical pleasure and emotional closeness, as well as sexual communication and intimacy.

5. If the exercise elicits significant emotional distress or couples find that they have a great deal of difficulty communicating during the exercise, professional counseling can often assist in resolving the interfering issues.

Women and men report that diminished libido is frequently associated with a decrease in sexual fantasies. Diminished libido can sometimes be stimulated by increasing sexual imagery and fantasy. Historically, most sexual literature, videos, and magazines have been developed to appeal to a male rather than female audience. Recently, however, some sexual videos are being marketed to appeal to couples and women. They typically include fewer close-ups of genitals during orgasm and have more emotional and romantic content and imagery. (See Recommended Resources at the end of the chapter). When libido is partially intact but difficulty sustaining arousal and/or having orgasms occurs, sharing sexual fantasies or watching sexually-oriented videos together may help sustain arousal. Similarly, introducing new kinds of sexual play into sexual behavior can help maintain arousal and trigger orgasms.

⊙ Erectile problems

TREATMENT OF PRIMARY sexual dysfunction in men frequently addresses erectile problems. A complex series of nerve impulses, which travel between the brain, spinal cord, and penis, initiate and maintain an erection. Accompanying these signals is an increase in the arterial blood flow to the corpus cavernosa (three cylinder-like areas of spongy tissue in the penis), causing these tissues to expand. The arterial inflow of blood, in association with relaxation of smooth muscle in the penis, compresses small veins through which blood normally exits the penis. This venous compression traps the blood in the penis and causes an erection. When nerve transmission is impaired, a man's ability to achieve or maintain an erection can be affected.

The lower (sacral) area of the spinal cord has nerve pathways traveling to and from the genitals, which allow for reflex erections. Reflex erections that do not involve the middle or upper parts of the spinal cord or brain can usually be triggered by stimulating the penis and scrotum directly. Therefore, some men who have impaired erectile function can obtain reflex erections by vigorously stimulating the penis and scrotum with a vibrator. Reflex erections can also result from "stuffing." To engage in stuffing, the woman sits astride her partner and inserts the flaccid penis into the (well-lubricated) vagina. Even if a reflex erection does not result from this motion, it frequently produces pleasurable sensations for both partners. However, stuffing must be done in a gentle fashion. The flaccid penis can fold back on itself and become squeezed by the pressure of the partner's weight, which can cause injury to the penis. In the presence of reduced sensation, the damage can go undetected because it occurs inside the penis.

Several options are available for treating erectile problems caused by MS.

Oral medications

Oral medicines known as phosphdiesterase type 5 inhibitors, or PDE-5 inhibitors (e.g., sildenafil citrate—Viagra®; vardenafil—Levitra®; and tadalafil—Cialis®) are used to help with erectile dysfunction. PDE-5 inhibitors work by blocking a chemical in erectile tissues that causes erections to become flaccid, which in turn allows for enhanced erections. In controlled clinical trials, all three of these medicines were associated with significantly improved erectile function and greater frequency of intercourse among men with impotence, whether the impotence was related to physical causes, psychological issues, or both.

All three of the medications are approved by the Food and Drug

Administration (FDA) for the treatment of erectile dysfunction in men. Of the three drugs, however, only Viagra® (the first of these drugs to arrive on the market) has been specifically tested in men with MS. In a placebo-controlled clinical trial of Viagra® in men with MS, Viagra® was shown to have a positive impact on quality of life—including sexual life, partnerships, family life, social contacts, and overall satisfaction. While all three of these medications have been used successfully by men with MS, they do not work for everyone.

The PDE-5 inhibitors, which take 30 minutes to an hour to become effective in the body, vary somewhat in the length of time they remain effective—ranging from a couple of hours to 36 hours. During this period of time, the man is able to achieve an erection in *response to appropriate erotic stimulation*. In the absence of stimulation, no erection will occur. While these medications enhance erectile function in men with erectile disturbances, they do not improve or increase sexual desire or resolve conflicts or tension within a relationship. Counseling is recommended to help restore intimacy and improve communication for those who have been experiencing significant relationship issues.

Since all PDE-5 inhibitors work with the same biochemical pathway, the precautions and side effects for the three drugs are similar. None are to be used by men who are taking nitrate-based medications (e.g., ISMO®, Imdur®, Nitro-Dur®, Nitro-Paste®, Nitrostat®, Nitro-Bid®, etc.) because the combination may cause a sudden and potentially dangerous reduction in blood pressure, *even if the nitrate medications are used only occasionally*. PDE-5 inhibitors cause a small transient decrease in blood pressure in most men. Coupled with the cardiovascular stress of intercourse, this side effect can cause heart attacks or strokes in men with pre-existing vascular disease. Men with recent heart attacks, significant high blood pressure, and/or heart disease should have a cardiology evaluation prior to starting on any of these medications. While it may be tempting to order one of these medications over the Internet, it is extremely important to consult with a physician before doing so.

Side effects of these medicines in the clinical trials were relatively infrequent, with headache, facial flushing, indigestion, dizziness, nasal congestion, and blue-green visual aura being reported. Priapism (overly prolonged erection) has also been reported as a rare side effect. In a normal erection, the penis remains rigid because the trapping mechanism keeps blood from flowing out of the penis until ejaculation occurs. This blockage of blood flow prevents the penis from receiving fresh oxygen for the period of time that the penis remains erect. Therefore, a man whose penis remains erect for too long a period of time risks irreversible damage to the erectile mechanism and to the penis itself. If a man's erection lasts longer than four hours, he must seek immediate medical treatment, since an erection lasting longer than 24 hours will permanently damage penile tissue.

All of the PDE-5 inhibitor medications are relatively expensive, and some insurance companies in the United States will not reimburse for the costs of these medications.

In addition to the PDE-5 inhibitors, there are other oral medicines in development for erectile dysfunction that work by enhancing or blocking chemical pathways in the brain and spinal cord that are related to sexual function. None of these have been tried to date in MS.

Medications administered by injection

Non-oral pharmacologic treatment of erectile dysfunction involves injecting medications into the penis to stimulate erections. This approach is typically used when oral medicines have not been effective. Unlike the oral medications that require erotic stimulation for an erection to occur, the injectable medications used in MS produce an erection regardless of the presence or absence of erotic stimulation. Although many men object to the idea of injecting medication into the penis to simulate erections, the injection is done with a very fine needle into an area at the base of the penis that is relatively insensitive to pain. Men who are particularly resistant to the idea of self-injecting can use an "-auto-injector" that works with a simple push-button mechanism. Most men report very little, if any, pain from this injection. The sensation is best described as similar to being flicked by a rubber band.

Three different injectable medications are commonly prescribed, and several others are under investigation. Prostaglandin E1 (alprostadil; Prostin VR®) has been approved by the FDA for the management of erectile problems and is the one used most commonly in MS. This vasodilator and smooth muscle relaxant is the natural substance released by the smooth muscle cells in the penis when a man is sexually excited. Relaxation of smooth muscle in the penis prevents blood from leaving the penis once it enters, allowing erection to occur.

The FDA has also approved alprostadil for use via urethral suppository (MUSE®). In this approach, a small plastic applicator inserts the drug into the urethra. The drug is absorbed into penile tissues and stimulates a satisfactory erection in most men who have erectile dysfunction. Approximately one-third of men report some penile discomfort with its use, and priapism can occur in rare instances.

Another drug used for injections, papaverine, is also a smooth muscle relaxant. Papaverine is infrequently associated with pain and is thus a good alternative for any men who experience discomfort with prostaglandin E1. Papaverine has a slightly greater tendency to cause scarring at the injection site. Because papaverine also remains active in the body for a somewhat longer period of time, it is associated with a greater risk of priapism. Although it is commonly prescribed, papaverine has not been approved by the FDA for the treatment of erectile dysfunction.

Phentolamine (Regitine® in the United States; Rogitine® in Canada) is sometimes used in combination with either prostaglandin E1 and/or papaverine to heighten their effectiveness. Phentolamine is an alpha-adrenergic blocking agent and will not induce erections without the presence of another medication (most frequently prostaglandin E1 and/or papaverine). Depending on the type of symptoms the man is experiencing; his physician may prescribe different combinations of these medications.

Priapism is a potential side effect of any of these treatments, particularly if too much medication is administered. Priapism almost never occurs in individuals who adhere to the prescribed dose of medication and who are properly trained in the injection procedures.

A second potential side effect of penile injections, which is experienced by approximately 7-10% of individuals, is scarring at the injection site. This problem very seldom occurs in men who have been properly trained in correct injection techniques. When scarring does occur, it takes the form of a small nodule in the subcutaneous tissue of the penis. Any man who is self-injecting should be examined by a physician every 3 months for possible scarring. These nodules typically disappear after the injections are stopped.

Penile prosthesis

Men who do not respond satisfactorily to oral medications or self-injection medications may find the surgically-implanted prosthesis to be a more satisfactory alternative. Following a careful evaluation of a man's history and presenting symptoms (medical, psychological, neurologic, and sexual), the physician will work with the person to determine which type of treatment would be most beneficial. A spouse or long-term sexual partner should be included in the decision to get an implant, as well as in the selection of the type of prosthesis to be used.

There are two types of penile prostheses—semirigid and inflatable. With the semirigid type, a flexible rod is implanted by a urologic surgeon in each of the erection chambers (corpus cavernosa) of the penis. These rods can be bent upward when an erection is desired and bent downward at other times. Following insertion of the rods, the penis remains somewhat enlarged, with a permanent semierection.

With the inflatable type of prosthesis, an erection is created by fluid that is pumped from a reservoir into balloons inserted in the corpus cavernosa. The fluid is pumped into the chambers when an erection is desired and transferred back to the reservoir when it is no longer wanted. The reservoir is surgically implanted behind the abdominal wall; the pump is implanted in the man's scrotum. Silicon tubing is used to connect the reservoir, pump, and balloons. Because the pump is inserted through a single, relatively invisible incision in the scrotum, this type of prosthesis is barely noticeable. However, operating the pump through the scrotum wall can be difficult for individuals who have reduced hand sensation or strength.

Extensive presurgery consultation with a urologist or a physician who is familiar with MS will help to ensure that the man and his partner have realistic expectations after the surgery. Research has shown that upward of 80% of men (and their partners) who use these types of prostheses find them satisfactory. Many men experience normal erectile sensations and normal orgasm. In addition, they are able to have an erection for as long as they choose to do so.

Complications associated with penile implants include those associated with surgery in general (i.e., problems with anesthesia and bleeding). Infection occurs in approximately 2-8% of men who receive prostheses and can be quite serious. In the event of infection, the entire device must be removed. Replacement of the implant following treatment of the infection is usually feasible, but often more complicated. A penile prosthesis is only recommended when less invasive efforts to manage erectile dysfunction are not successful. In other words, a man would be considered a candidate for a prosthesis only if noninvasive measures were unsuccessful, if he were unable to self-inject, or if an effective dosage level or combination of medications could not be found.

Non-medical/non-surgical interventions

A method for enhancing erections without the use of medicine or surgery involves the vacuum erection device (VED). The VED, which consists of a vacuum tube and constriction band, can be purchased with a prescription from a urologist or other MS physician. With the VED, a plastic tube is fitted over the flaccid penis, and a hand pump or suction tube is operated to create a vacuum. The vacuum draws blood into the erectile tissues and produces an erection, which is similar to the natural erectile process. Once engorgement of the penis is achieved, a latex band is slipped from the base of the cylinder onto the base of the penis. Air is returned to the cylinder, and the tube is removed. The band maintains engorgement of the penis by restricting venous return of blood to the body, thus allowing for intercourse or other sexual activity. The use of the band must be limited to 30 minutes or less to avoid any medical complications. Moderate hand sensation and dexterity are required for placing and removing the band in some models. Other models have assister sleeves that permit hands-free placement of the constriction band. For men who can attain erections readily but have difficulty maintaining them, the constriction band alone can be used with satisfactory results. Although minor side effects (e.g., skin irritation and bruising) are common, patient and partner satisfaction with a VED has been found to be high.

A number of other sexual aids, available by mail-order, do not require a physician's prescription (see mail order catalogues listed). Strap-on latex penises, some of which are hollow and can hold a flaccid or semierect penis, are preferred by some. Strap-on, battery-operated vibrators in the shape of a penis are also available.

Choosing a sexual device to aid with erections is best done with the advice of a urologist or sex therapist familiar with MS. If the man has a long-term sex partner, it is very important to include this person in the discussion. This will decrease anxiety and uncertainty when the devices are used and can enhance intimacy by allowing both sex partners to explore together. If there are struggles in communicating or if the partners feel inhibited about talking through these issues, counseling with a mental health professional who is knowledgeable about MS can facilitate the process.

The efficacy of any treatment depends on the ability of both partners to communicate openly about sexual issues and decide on methods that are comfortable and enjoyable for both. Education about treatment options provides people with MS and their partners with the language and knowledge that enables discussion and informed decision making.

Secondary Sexual Dysfunction In MS (Resulting From Other MS Symptoms)

IN MULTIPLE SCLEROSIS (MS), the incidence of fatigue, muscle tightness or spasms, bladder and bowel dysfunction, and pain, burning, or other discomfort can have adverse effects on the experience of sexual activity. The interference of these symptoms with sexual function can often be alleviated by taking an aggressive approach to symptom management. A significant part of managing secondary sexual dysfunction is to become well educated about the nature, causes, and treatments of those MS symptoms that affect sexual functioning.

◉ Fatigue

ONE OF THE most common secondary sexual symptoms in MS is fatigue. Fatigue greatly interferes with sexual desire and the physical ability to initiate and sustain sexual activity. Fatigue can be managed in a number of ways. It is often helpful to set aside time in the morning for sexual activity, since this is usually when MS fatigue is at its lowest ebb. Energy conservation techniques (e.g., taking naps and using a motorized scooter or other ambulation aids) can preserve the energy needed for sexual activities. Choosing sexual activities and positions that are less physically demanding or weight-bearing for the partner with MS may minimize fatigue during sex. In addition, a physician can prescribe a medication such as modafinil (Provigil®) or amantadine to help minimize fatigue. As you try to initiate some of these changes in your sexual life, be aware that they require open communication and a willingness to engage in some trial-and-error exploration. If you or your sexual partner find it difficult to communicate about alternatives, counseling may be helpful.

◉ Bladder and bowel symptoms

PHARMACOLOGIC INTERVENTIONS HAVE also been used to manage bladder and bowel symptoms in MS. Some common symptoms of bladder dysfunction include incontinence, urgency, and frequent urination. Anticholinergic medications help manage incontinence by reducing spasms of the bladder and the urethra. One side effect of bladder medications, however, is dryness of the vagina. As previously mentioned, vaginal dryness can be alleviated with generous amounts of a water-soluble lubricant (e.g., K-Y Jelly⁽ʳ⁾). A physician may be able to help modify daily medication schedules to maximize benefit and minimize negative side effects at the time of planned sexual activity.

Sexual interest is frequently inhibited by fear of bladder or bowel accidents during sexual activity. It is important for partners to openly discuss their concerns about incontinence with one another.

Most partners are willing to "take the chance" after they have been informed of the issues and educated about the measures that are being taken to manage the problem. By strategizing together, and with the healthcare team, couples can minimize the risk of incontinence during sexual activity, thereby increasing their relaxation and pleasure. The partner who has MS may need to tailor his or her symptomatic management strategies to allow for anticipated sexual activity. If, for example, a person is taking anticholinergic medications for bladder storage dysfunction, it may be advisable to take the medication 30 minutes before anticipated sexual activity in order to minimize bladder contractions. Because these medicines increase vaginal dryness, a woman may need to compensate by using a water-soluble lubricant. Restricting fluid intake for an hour or two before sex and conducting intermittent catheterization just before sexual activity will also minimize incontinence. For men who are concerned about small amounts of urinary leakage, wearing a condom during sex is advised.

If an indwelling catheter is used, healthcare providers may be able to offer tips for handling or temporarily removing catheters. If a woman needs to keep the catheter in place, she can move it out of the way by folding it over and taping it to her stomach with paper tape. It is a good idea to experiment with different sexual positions and activities to find those that feel the most comfortable with the catheter in place. The book *Choices: A Guide to Sex Counseling with Physically Disabled Adults* (see Additional Readings at the end of the chapter) offers illustrations of positions for sexual intercourse that are most beneficial for managing catheters and a wide range of physical limitations. Many people put a plastic mattress pad on the bed and keep towels handy to wipe up any leaks or accidents.

The fear of losing bladder or bowel control during sexual activity, or feeling that one is unattractive because of MS-related equipment or physical symptoms, can inhibit sexual desire and increase feelings of vulnerability and anxiety. Having frank and open discussions with a sexual partner about bladder or bowel dysfunction before engaging in sexual activity may remove some of the fear about losing control and allow for a more enjoyable sexual experience.

⊙ Spasticity

SPASTICITY CAN MAKE straightening the legs, or changing leg positions for sexual activity, quite painful. Active symptomatic management of spasticity will minimize its impact on sexuality. Range of motion and other physical therapy exercises are commonly employed, as well as antispasticity medications, such as baclofen and tizanidine (Zanaflex®.) Exploring alternative sexual positions for intercourse is helpful when spasticity is a problem. Women who have spasticity of the adductor muscles may find it difficult or painful to separate their legs. Changing positions (e.g., lying on one side with the partner approaching from behind) to accommodate this symptom may be important. Taking an antispasticity medication 30 minutes before anticipated sexual activity can be helpful. Be sure, however, to discuss any medication changes with your physician.

⊙ Weakness

WEAKNESS IS A common MS symptom that frequently necessitates finding new positions for satisfactory sexual activities. Reclining (non–weight-bearing) positions do not place as much strain on muscles and are therefore less tiring. Pillows can be used to improve positioning and reduce muscle strain. Inflatable wedge-shaped pillows (available by mail order) are specifically designed to provide back support during sexual activity. Oral sex requires less movement than intercourse, and using a hand-held or strap-on vibrator can help compensate for hand weakness while providing sexual stimulation.

⊙ Pain and other discomforts

OTHER SECONDARY SEXUAL symptoms may include pain, tingling or burning sensations, and positional discomfort. These symptoms can interfere with intimacy and sexuality by making it difficult to enjoy sexual activities or find comfortable sexual positions. Tingling and burning sensations can sometimes be relieved by an antiepileptic drug such as gabapentin (Neuronton®), carbamazepine (Tegretol®), or divalproex sodium

(Depakote®), or by an antidepressant such as amitriptyline (Elavil®). Anxieties about hurting a sex partner are fairly common when there are significant changes in physical functioning. Education and discussion about MS symptoms will enable partners to air concerns while planning for sexual encounters. Conducting a "positioning exercise" before sex is attempted will help determine if the new positions are comfortable and feasible without introducing anxiety during sexual activity.

⊙ Distractibility

SUSTAINED ATTENTION AND myotonia (increasing muscle tension) are usually required for sexual feelings to build progressively toward orgasm. MS can cause impairment of attention and concentration that may interfere with maintaining sexual desire during sexual activities (see Chapter 6). This may, in turn, lead to feelings of rejection or inadequacy in the partner and guilt in the person with MS. Accepting distractibility as a valid MS symptom and discussing ways to help compensate for it are crucial steps toward finding a solution.

Attention and/or concentration problems tend to be worse when a person is fatigued, so evaluating the person's fatigue level and compensating accordingly are vitally important. The main strategy to deal with distractibility is to minimize nonsexual stimuli and maximize sensual and sexual stimuli. Creating a romantic mood and setting, using sensual music and lighting, talking in sexy ways, and engaging in erotic touching provide multisensory stimuli that minimize "cognitive drift" during sex. Introducing humor at those moments when the person "loses attention" allows mutual acceptance of this frustrating symptom and helps minimize its impact.

In summary, there are several approaches to managing secondary sexual problems in MS. First, it is important to become familiar with the MS symptoms and treatments that affect sexual functioning. Information can be obtained directly from physicians, nurses, or other health professionals who are involved in the care of people with MS, or from MS literature.

In addition, a wealth of knowledge can be found by speaking casually with others via MS chat rooms and bulletin boards on the Internet or through local support groups and other activities run by and for individuals who have MS. Information about support groups, the Internet, and other MS-related information can be found by contacting your chapter of the Multiple Sclerosis Society in the United States or Canada or the office of the International Federation of Multiple Sclerosis Societies in London, England.

Second, it may be helpful to utilize various pharmacologic approaches in managing secondary sexual dysfunction. A physician who is competent in the care of individuals with MS may be able to prescribe medications to alleviate the symptoms that hinder sexual enjoyment. In addition, a physician can help modify treatment regimens to best accommodate sexual needs.

Last, planning for intimacy and modifying sexual activities can be quite beneficial. Although planning for sexual activity may initially take away some of the romance and spontaneity, it will eventually lead to a more positive, satisfying sexual experience.

Planning for intimate activity and altering familiar sexual behaviors can sometimes be emotionally frightening or uncomfortable. It is easier to adapt to these modifications by having open communication and flexibility within the relationship. Counseling can be helpful in maintaining intimacy by assisting couples to discuss these issues with one another and encouraging the exploration of new approaches to intimate and sexual communication.

Tertiary Sexual Dysfunction In MS
(Related To Psychological, Social, And Cultural Issues)

THE PHYSICAL CHANGES experienced by people who have MS can alter their view of themselves as sexual beings, as well as their perception of the way others view them. The psychological and cultural context in which physical changes occur can adversely affect self-image, mood, sexual and intimate desire, and the ease or difficulty with which people with MS communicate with their partners.

☉ Self-image and body image

IN WESTERN SOCIETIES, women are particularly susceptible to having a negative body image. The media's depiction of women as unrealistically thin and oozing with sensuality is at odds with the reality of most women's personal experience. The extremely high prevalence of diagnosed eating disorders, the variety of commercially-packaged diet programs and cosmetic surgery centers, and the multi-billion-dollar cosmetics industry targeting women, all reflect the efforts of women to reconcile their sensual and sexual self-image with the unrealistic cultural feminine mystique. Women with MS may have difficulty enjoying their sensual and sexual nature because of the gap between their internalized cultural images of the "sensual woman" and their MS-related physical changes.

Similar cultural pressures affect men. Internalized cultural images of men as potent, aggressive, and powerful are at odds with the illness experience. MS-associated changes in erectile capacity or employment can be associated with an internal sense of failure or defectiveness as the discrepancy between culturally induced self-expectations and one's personal experience grows wide.

☉ Changing roles

CHANGES IN FAMILY and societal roles secondary to disability can affect one's capacity for intimacy and sexuality. The person with MS who has difficulty fulfilling his or her designated work and household roles may no longer feel like an equal partner. The partner of a severely disabled individual may feel overburdened by additional care giving, household, and employment responsibilities (see Chapter 9). Their intimate relationship can be threatened by the growing tension that results from these feelings.

In addition, the care giving partner (either male or female) may have trouble switching from the nurturant role of caregiver to the more sensual role of lover. As a sexual partner of a woman (or man) with a disability, a man may begin to think of his partner as too fragile or easily injured, or as a "patient" who is ill and therefore unable to be sexually expressive. If it is practical or culturally acceptable, having nonfamily members perform care giving activities helps minimize this role conflict. When care giving must be performed by the sexual partner, separating care giving activities from times that are dedicated to romantic and sexual activities can minimize this conflict.

Accompanying these role changes may be an increasing sense of isolation in the relationship and less understanding of the partner's struggles and perspectives. The diminishing capacity to understand and work through these issues creates greater isolation and misunderstanding, leading to increasing resentments.

⊙ Cultural expectations regarding sexual behavior

THE RELIGIOUS, CULTURAL, and societal influences in our lives help shape our thoughts, views, and expectations about sexuality. One of the notions about sexuality that prevails in Western culture is a "goal-oriented" approach to sex. In this approach, the sexual activity is done with the goal of having penile-vaginal intercourse, ultimately leading to orgasm. Here, the sexual behaviors labeled as foreplay (e.g., erotic conversations, touching, kissing, and genital stimulation) are seen as steps that inevitably lead to intercourse rather than as physically and emotionally satisfying sexual activities in their own right. Hence, couples are not thought to be having "real" sex until they are engaging in coitus, and sex is typically not considered "successfully completed" until orgasm occurs.

This Western view of sexuality leads to spending a great deal of time and energy worrying about the MS-related barriers to intercourse and orgasm ("the goal") rather than seizing the opportunity to explore physically and emotionally satisfying alternatives to intercourse. The capacity to discover new and fulfilling ways to compensate for sexual limitations requires that couples be able to let go of preconceived notions of what sex should be and focus instead on openly communicating their sexual needs and pleasures without fear of ridicule or embarrassment.

⊙ MS-related emotional challenges

THE MS EXPERIENCE is frequently associated with emotional challenges, including grief, demoralization, and sometimes clinical depression (see Chapter 2). These emotional struggles may temporarily dampen interest in sex or the ability to give and receive sexual pleasure. Coping with emotional changes to enhance sexuality has several aspects: assessment, education, professional treatment, and coping interventions. Assessment of clinical depression can be done by a mental health professional who is familiar with MS. Treatment that involves antidepressant medications and psychotherapy typically offers symptom relief, including the restoration of sexual interest. (Because loss of libido and orgasmic changes are common side effects of some antidepressant medications, it is important to discuss medication options thoroughly with your physician.)

Changes in self-esteem and body image are frequently associated with the losses imposed by chronic illness. These changes are accompanied by a normal grieving process that tends to ebb and flow over the course of the disease. In addition, the demanding and unpredictable course of MS can lead to stress and anxiety, which, in turn, set the stage for partners to "take out" MS-related frustrations on each other or emotionally withdraw from the relationship. The times when partners need the most support and encouragement from each other are precisely the times when it may be most difficult to offer that help. Education about the emotional challenges in MS and approaches to dealing with them is available through the National MS Society (see Chapter 12).

⊙ The role of effective communication

ONE OF THE most important coping interventions in dealing with body image and emotional changes is ongoing, effective, intimate communication with one's long-term sexual partner. If the long-term relationship represents an important context of sexuality, communication skills constitute the vehicle of sexual expression. Exploring new options, discussing disappointments, and expressing what partners feel and want may be particularly difficult in the face of coping with all the other changes associated with MS. MS peer groups, couples groups, and/or individual or couples counseling can facilitate the communication process.

There are several fundamental components of successful communication. The first is *active listening*, which encompasses such behaviors as giving undivided attention, observing each other's body language, fully hearing each other's messages before responding, and requesting clarification if necessary. When these skills are developed, partners are more capable of offering *empathy*, which is one of the most crucial interpersonal skills needed to enhance and maintain a harmonious and pleasurable relationship. Empathic communication requires that an individual be able to comprehend his or her partner's thoughts and feelings in a given situation *and* be able to convey the understanding to that person. There is a greater chance of enhancing emotional intimacy, even at difficult moments, if both partners feel there is mutual understanding and respect.

Talking with Healthcare Providers and Acquiring Information

OFTEN, NEUROLOGISTS AND other MS healthcare providers do not spontaneously bring up the subject of sexuality. They may ignore sexuality because they perceive this line of questioning as an unwelcome intrusion into their patients' private lives, because they are personally uncomfortable asking about sexuality, or because they lack professional training in this area. Although it can be difficult and potentially embarrassing, your sexuality is important enough for you to bring up with your primary MS physician. Discuss your changes in sexual feelings and ask directly about treatments that are available to enhance sexuality. If you have a sexual partner, bring your partner with you or share the information. Ask your doctor about how your symptoms and the medications used to treat them may be affecting your sexual response. Although the burden of opening the door to communication about sexuality may initially fall on you, taking this step with your healthcare team will ensure that this frequently untreated symptom receives the attention it deserves.

ADDITIONAL READINGS

National MS Society Publications
(available by calling 1-800-FIGHT-MS (1-800-344-4867) or
online at http://www.nationalmssociety.org/library.asp)
MS and Intimacy.

GENERAL READINGS

Kaufman M, Silverberg C, Odette F. *The Ultimate Guide to Sex and Disability.*
San Francisco: Cleis Press, 2003.

Kroll K, Klein EL. *Enabling romance: A guide to love, sex, and relationships for the
disabled (and the people who care about them).* Bethesda, MD: Woodbine
House, 1995.

Neistadt ME, Freda M. *Choices: A guide to sex counseling with physically disabled
adults.* Malabar, FL: Robert E. Krieger Publishing Co., 1987.

Winks C, Semans A. *The Good Vibrations Guide to Sex* (3rd ed.) San
Francisco: Cleis Press.

ONLINE RESOURCE

www.goodvibes.com —Good Vibrations is a California-based
company with three physical locations, a website, and paper
catalog. The website contains disability-related information as
well as an online magazine that features a regular column about
sex and disability.

5

Fertility, Pregnancy, and Childbirth

Kathy Birk, M.D.
Barbara Giesser, M.D.

FAMILY PLANNING, PREGNANCY, and childrearing are major life events for many couples, deeply embedded in their ongoing evolution as a family unit. The diagnosis of multiple sclerosis (MS) makes the choices and decisions that surround childbearing somewhat more complicated. The disease is often diagnosed during early adulthood, when individuals and couples are in the midst of major career and family decisions. By its very nature, MS adds to the usual uncertainty and unpredictability of life. Plans that had previously been taken for granted are suddenly called into question, and new fears and doubts can create a high degree of stress and anxiety.

Newly diagnosed individuals and their partners want to know how MS will affect their ability to have and raise children. The answer to this important question needs to be divided into two parts: one pertains to the immediate, short-term issues of planning, pregnancy, and childbirth, whereas the other pertains to those that are more relevant to the long-term issues of parenting and family stability. A more complete discussion of the parenting experience in MS can be found in Chapter 6.

Short-Term Issues

The Inheritability Of MS

POPULATION, FAMILY, AND twin studies suggest a genetic component in a person's susceptibility to developing MS. It has been estimated that children who have a parent with MS have approximately a 2-5/100 (about 3.0%) risk of developing MS. Because the lifetime risk of MS in the general population is approximately 1/750 (0.1%), this means that the child of a parent with MS has a 30 times greater risk of developing the disease. Although couples wishing to have children need to be aware of the increased risk, it is also important for them to bear in mind that the risk factor remains relatively small.

Fertility

FERTILITY IS, FOR the most part, unaffected by MS. This means that couples must make the same decisions regarding birth control as do individuals without neurologic problems. Any form of birth control is permissible with MS; choices should be made on the basis of ease and effectiveness. A woman who is experiencing weakness or tremor in her hands may find it difficult to insert a diaphragm. Similarly, a man might find a condom too cumbersome. However, the sexual partner can learn to insert a diaphragm or put on the condom and make this an enjoyable part of sexual foreplay.

Oral contraceptives are a safe and effective option; they have not been shown to increase the risk of developing MS or to affect the disease course following diagnosis. The intrauterine device (IUD) is also an acceptable alternative, but its effectiveness and safety may be compromised by the long-term use of antibiotics or immunosuppressive drugs that can lower a woman's resistance to infection. The copper IUD currently available in the United States is 98-99% effective and safe. Once inserted by the physician (during an outpatient visit), IUDs can be used safely for a period of 5-10 years without being changed, depending on the type that is used.

Although MS does not have any negative impact on a woman's fertility, the erectile and/or orgasmic difficulties that some men experience as a result of MS can interfere with fertility (see Chapter 4 for a discussion of sexuality in MS). It is important for young couples in the family planning stage to be aware that the occurrence of these erectile and orgasmic problems depends on the location of the MS plaques and is unrelated to the man's age or to the length of time that he has had MS.

A variety of options are now available for the treatment of erectile problems. These are discussed in Chapter 4. Problems with orgasm, which have been reported in a series of surveys by 44-77% of men with MS, may also respond to treatment. "Dry orgasms" occur when there is an absence of seminal emission or when semen is ejaculated in retrograde (backward) fashion into the bladder. Since either of these would impair fertility, men with dry orgasms who wish to have a child should not hesitate to speak to their physician. Treatments involving medication and/or electroejaculation have proved beneficial with these types of orgasmic difficulties.

It is important to keep in mind that couples with or without MS can experience infertility problems at any time, even if they have already had a child. The co-existence of MS should not interfere with a thorough infertility evaluation. Both members of the couple should be evaluated because 40% of infertility problems involve the male partner. A variety of treatments are available to assist with infertility problems. In addition, adoption remains a viable (although potentially costly) way to build a family.

How MS Affects Pregnancy And Childbirth

MS does not appear to affect the course of pregnancy, labor, or delivery. There is no increased risk of spontaneous abortions, labor or delivery complications, fetal malformations, or stillbirths. Therefore, couples do not need to be concerned that the mother's MS will affect her ability to have a normal, healthy baby.

Anesthetics That Are Safe For Use During Labor Or Cesarean Section

Epidural anesthesia is considered safe and effective for pain relief during labor as well as for surgery, in the event that a cesarean section is required. It is thought to be safer than spinal anesthesia, which has traditionally been avoided in all individuals who have MS. Although general anesthesia is considered safe for women who require cesarean section, most women seem to prefer an epidural anesthesia.

Medications That Are Safe For Use During Pregnancy

IDEALLY, WOMEN SHOULD seek medical advice *before conception* in order to review medications they are currently using, eliminate anything that is unnecessary, and substitute safer drugs where appropriate. While there are some medications that can safely be used during pregnancy without harm to the developing fetus, the recommended strategy is to review everything you are taking (both prescription and non-prescription) with your healthcare provider and take only those medications that have been specifically prescribed and/or approved for use during pregnancy. A woman who is taking medications and becomes pregnant should review those medications with her physician as soon as possible.

In particular, the disease-modifying medications—interferon beta 1a (Avonex® and Rebif®), interferon beta 1b (Betaseron®), and glatiramer acetate (Copaxone®)—are not approved for use during pregnancy. The beta interferon medications (Avonex, Betaseron, and Rebif) have all been given a Category C rating by the FDA, indicating that they have been shown in animal studies to increase the risk of miscarriage. Copaxone has a Category B rating, meaning that no harm has been demonstrated in animal studies, but there are no data in humans to demonstrate their safety. Fortunately, these immunomodulating medications are not as critical during pregnancy because the hormones produced naturally by the woman's body during this time provide a similar degree of protection. Pregnancy-related hormones work to reduce immune activity in order to prevent the mother's body from rejecting the "foreign" fetus. Because a fertilized egg begins to develop well before a woman knows she is pregnant, it is recommended that women stop their disease-modifying medication at least 1-2 menstrual cycles before trying to conceive. The medication can be resumed immediately after delivery if the woman chooses not to breast-feed her baby.

Mitoxantrone (Novantrone®) and other chemotherapeutic agents that are sometimes prescribed in MS (e.g., cyclophosphamide, methotrexate, azathioprine) are all Category D or X, indicating that they are known to harm a developing fetus. Women are advised to take a pregnancy test prior to taking any of these medications and avoid becoming pregnant while taking them.

MS And Breast-Feeding

WOMEN WHO WISH to nurse are encouraged to do so, provided that they have the requisite strength and stamina to manage the baby safely and do not require medications that would make nursing inadvisable. Breast-feeding has not been found to be associated with any change in the likelihood, timing, or severity of postpartum MS exacerbations.

For the first several weeks post partum, an infant should nurse every 2-4 hours in order to stimulate the growth of the mother's milk supply. Feedings can be at more frequent intervals during the day and every 4 hours during the night to allow the mother more extended periods of sleep. If at all possible, she should remain in bed for the nighttime feedings and let her partner (or another helper) bring the baby to her and then put the baby back to bed when the feeding is finished. Once the milk supply is well established, a breast pump can be used during the day to supply milk to be given by bottle at night. As an alternative, formula can be used for night feedings when the infant is approximately 2-3 weeks of age, after the mother has established her milk supply.

Because fatigue may adversely affect milk production, it is important for a new mother to have at least 8 hours of bed rest at night, rest time during the day, and sufficient help. Because these demands can rest quite heavily on a working father, creative predelivery planning is required to try to meet everyone's needs.

Many of the disease-modifying and symptom management drugs prescribed for MS are not recommended or approved for use during breast-feeding because they can pass into the breast

---

milk and affect the baby. Since the choice to breast-feed means that a woman cannot resume taking her disease-modifying medication (Avonex®, Betaseron®, Copaxone®, or Rebif®), she should discuss the relative risks and benefits with her physician. A woman whose MS was particularly active prior to pregnancy, or who experienced an attack during the pregnancy, might determine with her doctor that resuming her medication as soon as possible would be the best course of action. Another woman, whose disease has been relatively inactive, might decide to delay resuming her medication for as long as she chooses to breast-feed her baby. This is one of those situations for which there are no definitive answers. The choice is a very personal one, to be made after open and honest discussion with one's physician.

How Pregnancy And Childbirth Affect MS

BEFORE 1950, VIRTUALLY all published literature and medical opinion advised women with MS against becoming pregnant. It was believed that pregnancy would worsen the woman's MS, eventually making it impossible for her to parent effectively. Beginning in 1950, all evidence started to point in a different direction. Several studies were published presenting retrospective reports of women with MS who had given birth. Taken together, these studies examined more than 925 pregnancies. Only 10% of the women experienced any worsening of their MS during pregnancy, whereas 29% experienced temporary worsening of the disease within 6 months after delivery.

In 1998, a European study of 254 women and 269 pregnancies reported a 70% decline in exacerbation rate during the last trimester of pregnancy (an effect that is more than twice that of the current disease-modifying therapies, each of which reduces the relapse rate by about 30%). During the first three months after delivery, women experienced a rebound 70% increase in relapse rate before returning to their pre-pregnancy baseline relapse rate.

These findings have now been confirmed in several additional studies; the average expected rate of exacerbations in women decreases progressively over the course of pregnancy, indicating that certain pregnancy-associated hormones and immunoactive proteins protect a pregnant woman who has MS. Women generally report feeling better during their pregnancies than they felt before becoming pregnant. As a result of these findings, the pregnancy hormone estriol (a form of estrogen) is now being actively studied as a potential treatment for women with MS.

In addition, a retrospective study of 178 women with MS found no difference in long-term disability levels of women who had experienced zero, one, or two or more pregnancies. The researchers concluded that the number of pregnancies has no effect on a woman's ultimate level of disability. This finding is difficult to interpret, however, because it is possible that women with more severe disease chose to have fewer pregnancies than did women with less severe disease.

In a Swedish study, researchers concluded that pregnancy had both short- and long-term effects on the course of MS. In addition to the expected decreased risk of exacerbation during pregnancy, their findings suggested that women who have gone through a pregnancy after the onset of MS might have a reduced risk of developing a progressive course of the disease.

In summary, studies have consistently shown that a woman's MS is likely to be stable, or even improved, during the actual 9 months of pregnancy. These studies offer some reassurance for women who are concerned about stopping their disease-modifying medication in order to become pregnant; the hormone produced during pregnancy offered at least as much protection as these medications. The risk of exacerbation following pregnancy has been found to range from 20-75% (regardless of whether the pregnancy goes to term or ends prematurely due to miscarriage or elective abortion). Most research supports the view that pregnancy does not affect the final course and degree of disability experienced by women with MS.

Long-Term Issues

THE LONG-TERM issues surrounding planning, pregnancy, and childbirth involve more complex questions and answers. Because MS is so unpredictable in its course and symptom picture, it is impossible for couples or their doctors to predict what the future will bring. Prospective parents with MS often ask whether they will be able to care for a child. Typically, they are picturing themselves attempting to hold, nurse, carry, or play with their new baby. Although these are important concerns, they are only the beginning; babies do not remain babies very long. The individual with MS and his or her partner need to consider the following: their financial and emotional security as a couple; their individual views of parenting; and their ability to handle major role shifts within the family if they become necessary.

Financial And Emotional Security

ALL PROSPECTIVE PARENTS, with or without the added complications of MS, need to assess their ability to provide a safe and secure environment for their children. Along with the joys children bring come additional pressures and responsibilities that can stress even the strongest relationship. A husband and wife who are already coping with MS need to think constructively about the future and plan defensively. Because it is impossible to predict the course of the disease, it is necessary to hope for the best while being prepared for whatever may occur (see Chapter 12 for a discussion of life planning). Thus, couples need to consider what they would do if the primary breadwinner became too disabled to work, how the children would be cared for if the primary caregiver became too disabled, and whether additional help and support would be available from the extended family. By discussing these issues honestly, couples can make more realistic decisions, reduce some of the stress of uncertainty, and feel more in control of their lives.

Parenting Style

INDIVIDUALS WITH MS often ask if they will be able to be good parents. The more important question is what being a "good parent" means to them. Whether they realize it or not, most people have an image of the kind of mother or father they want to be, and this image often involves very specific kinds of behaviors.

Men, for example, often think of fathering as playing sports, going camping, or roughhousing with the kids. "How can I be a good father if I can't even throw a baseball?" Women talk about being able to attend school functions, be a room-mother, carpool to various activities, and balance the demands of home and work. Both men and women express concerns about being able to maintain authority and discipline if they become disabled. Both worry about their ability to be good role models for their kids.

Couples who raise these important questions may want to begin thinking about parenting in a more flexible way. "Good" parenting can take many forms. The feelings that parents have for their children can be expressed in a variety of actions and activities. The ability to think more flexibly about parenting roles will relieve some of the pressure that prospective parents feel. Knowing that there is more than one way to do the job can make it easier to anticipate success. The confidence that parents have in their ability to provide love and nurturance will translate into feelings of confidence and security for their children (see Chapter 6 for further discussion of parenting issues).

Role Flexibility

OVER THE COURSE of their relationship, members of a couple gradually take shared or primary responsibility for certain roles (e.g., breadwinner, household manager, primary caregiver to the children, or financial planner). Sometimes this division of labor is done with much discussion and negotiation, and sometimes by tacit agreement with no real discussion or awareness of the decision-making process. However the process occurs, it is done in the face of an uncertain future. No couple knows for sure what the future will bring, but they hope and assume that it will happen as they have planned, with each able to carry out his or her chosen roles.

Couples who question whether it is wise for them to have children should think about how they would feel in the event that significant role changes became necessary. Would a man want to start a family if he knew that he might one day have to take over primary childrearing responsibilities? Would a woman want to start a family if she knew that she might have to become the sole breadwinner? There are no correct answers to these questions; each individual and each couple will respond differently. Once again, the ability to talk honestly about these questions will enable couples to make more realistic decisions and reduce future stress and resentment.

The Problem With Probability Statements

WHEN DISCUSSING WITH prospective parents their family planning decisions, professionals tend to fall back on statements of statistical probability: the likelihood of exacerbations; the likelihood of various disease outcomes; the likelihood of a child developing MS. Couples need to understand the meaning of these statistical statements. If a particular woman, for example, becomes one of the very few whose disease progresses unremittingly after childbirth, it does not matter to her that most other women do well. She will still have to cope with her situation. If one child in a family eventually develops MS, it does not matter to that family that the vast majority of children never develop the disease; the family will still have to cope. In making their family-planning decisions, couples would do well to think through the potential outcomes carefully so that they will feel more educated and prepared whatever the future brings.

Support For Families And Their Decisions

AS DIFFERENT COUPLES consider the various issues described here, they will come to a variety of conclusions. Some will make no change in their plans; others may decide not to have children or to begin their family but limit the size to smaller than they had originally planned; still others may decide to adopt a child instead of, or in addition to, having a child of their own. Many of these couples will experience some sense of loss as they reshape their dreams. Grieving over this kind of loss is a natural part of the gradual restructuring of a person's self-image and personal plans that necessarily accompanies chronic disease (see Chapter 2 for a discussion of the emotions in MS). It is important to recognize these feelings of sadness or loss for what they are, and seek counseling or other support if the need arises.

Similarly, those who proceed with their family plans only to discover that they are among the very few who run into major difficulties may find that this unexpected outcome can lead to feelings of anger, guilt, and anxiety. Couples do not need to handle these feelings alone, and they should feel free to seek assistance from a counselor or clergyman.

ADDITIONAL READINGS

National MS Society Publications

MS and Pregnancy—A reprint from the Society's magazine, InsideMS, available online in PDF format at http://www.nationalmssocie ty.org/pdf/Brochures/MSandPregnancy.pdf.

MS and Pregnancy—Part of the Society's Web Spotlight Series, available at http://www.nationalmssociety.org/spotlight-pregnancy.asp.

GENERAL READINGS

Birk K, Giesser B, Werner M. Fertility, pregnancy, childbirth, and gynecologic care. In: Kalb R, (ed.) Multiple Sclerosis: The Questions You Have—The Answers You Need (3rd ed). New York: Demos Medical Publishing, 2004.

6

Parenting Issues

Peggy Crawford, Ph.D., LISW
Deborah Miller, Ph.D.

THE POTENTIAL STRESSES associated with chronic illness, whether they are physical, psychological, social, or economic, affect not only the person diagnosed with the disease, but also other family members. This chapter discusses issues related to parenting and how the parent-child relationship can be affected when a parent has a chronic illness such as MS. Our emphasis is on supporting the normal development of both children and parents, and on enhancing individual and family abilities while minimizing their disabilities.

The various symptoms of MS are considered in relation to their potential impact on the emotional, social, and financial functioning of the family. In addition, some of the common responses of children to their parent's illness are described. Illness-related changes in the family unit and how they interact in an ongoing way with its pre-existing organizational and coping styles are considered.

The Impact of a Parent's Illness on Children

COMMON SENSE SUGGESTS that children who have a seriously ill parent would be at increased risk for physical, emotional, and social problems. Studies involving parental illnesses such as cancer, arthritis, diabetes, and chronic pain have shown that children who have chronically ill parents have significantly higher levels of emotional distress, behavioral problems, somatic (bodily) concerns, and lower levels of self-esteem and social competence than children who have physically healthy parents. Although parental illness thus appears to be associated with some difficulties in children's adjustment and functioning, the existing research is too limited and methodologically inadequate to provide firm conclusions about the relationships between specific types of illnesses and different aspects of children's social and emotional development. However, there is evidence for other factors that might affect this relationship, including the gender of the ill parent and the child; the age of the child; the child's conceptual understanding of the parent's illness; the quality of the relationship between the child and the well parent; the marital adjustment of the parents; and the mental health of both parents.

Only a few studies have specifically examined the relationship between a parent's MS and the adjustment of children in the family. Several early investigations reported some degree of emotional and social distress in these children, but more recent studies have reported no significant psychological or behavioral difficulties. In one of the few studies that compared these children to children of healthy, nondisabled parents, adolescents from families in which one of the parents had MS were found to be psychologically healthy, more sensitive to the needs of others, more self-reliant, and less likely to take life for granted than their peers. However, these adolescents were also significantly more worried about the health of both of their parents than were the teens in the control group.

How Do MS-Related Changes Affect the Parent–Child Relationship?

Physical Symptoms

PHYSICAL SYMPTOMS INCLUDE highly visible ones, such as walking problems or tremor, as well as those that are less visible, including severe fatigue, visual difficulties, and bladder and bowel problems. Most children have less difficulty understanding obvious symptoms that they see on a day-to-day basis. However, they may not understand that these symptoms do not necessarily "get better," like a cold or the flu, and that they may become more serious over time.

Symptoms that are less visible are generally more difficult for both children and adults to comprehend, and they are therefore more easily misinterpreted. For example, it is not unusual for a child to interpret a parent's fatigue as laziness or disinterest. After all, from a child's point of view, fatigue is easily remedied by a good night's sleep or a nap. Consider the following example. Sammy was a 10-year-old boy who aspired to be a pitcher for his hometown's baseball team. He often wanted to work on his skills by practicing after school with his father. Unfortunately, the late afternoon practice sessions coincided with his father's peak period of MS-related fatigue. Believing that his father spent all day resting since he no longer worked, Sammy began to accuse him of being lazy and not caring. His father used some creative problem-solving and suggested to Sammy that they get up half an hour earlier on school days to practice while it was still cool and he felt more rested.

Parents who have difficulty walking or using their arms and hands may find themselves limited in their ability to physically care for a young child. When this occurs, they may need to consider the difficult but sometimes necessary option of sharing care-taking responsibilities with others. The parent's primary goal in this situation should be to find someone who can be trusted to provide some of the hands-on care without undermining the parent's efforts or competing for the child's love and attention.

Mothers and fathers often worry about their ability to be "good parents" if they are physically unable to do things with their children that parents typically do (e.g., share a bike ride, walk them to school, or participate in sports). This inability to carry out some of the parenting activities that they had always pictured themselves doing with their children may cause intense feelings of sadness and loss. Although children may initially express disap-

pointment and even anger over the parent's inability to participate in some activities, they are often quite happy to have the parent present to observe their skills and offer support.

Parents should also enlist the help of family members and
friends whom they trust and with whom the child feels comfortable. Consider the following example. Ms. A was a single mother
who had a 7-year-old son. Because of her physical limitations,
she was unable to participate with him in the recreational activities at the neighborhood park. Her elderly parents with whom
they lived were not able to help, and her former husband only
visited his son on a very irregular basis. The young boy was disappointed and angry about missing out on these activities.
Ultimately, the mother enlisted the help of her unmarried brother,
who enjoyed spending time with his only nephew. The boy was
thrilled to have both an active companion *and* an enthusiastic spec-
tator going to the park with him.

Many mothers and fathers associate increasing disability with
increased limitations on their ability to discipline their children.
These parents tend to focus on the physical aspects of discipline
rather than on the necessary behavioral and communication skills,
such as communicating clear and consistent expectations and
consequences. Even with consistency, however, children sometimes challenge parents by "testing the limits" in order to reassure themselves that the parent is still in charge and can provide
the care they need.

Parents often find it helpful to identify other adults, with and
without MS, with whom they can share parenting concerns. MS
support groups and parenting workshops provide valuable opportunities for discussing parenting questions and developing a supportive social network of friends. Parenting workshops and
specialized group programs for parents with MS and their children are available in some communities through the National MS
Society or local MS treatment center (see Chapter 13).

Cognitive Impairment

LIKE OTHER INVISIBLE symptoms, cognitive symptoms associated with MS (see Chapter 2) may be particularly difficult for

children to understand. The most common cognitive impairments include problems with memory and concentration and an overall slowing of thought processes. Specific functions that are likely to be affected include learning and remembering new information, verbal fluency, maintaining attention for sustained periods (concentration), and executive functions (e.g., organizational and problem-solving). Children as well as adults frequently misinterpret these symptoms. For example, it is not unusual for a parent's forgetfulness to be interpreted as "not listening" or "not caring." As a result, the child feels hurt and angry and the parent feels frustrated and misunderstood. Children may begin to wonder if their parent is "becoming stupid," not paying attention, or simply not trying hard enough, especially when the parent has difficulty helping the child with homework.

Cognitive impairments can also interfere with usual parental responsibilities such as maintaining a child's schedule of appointments and activities. Consider the example of Stacy, who was angry and disappointed about missing an anticipated field trip with her fourth-grade class. Stacy's mother, whose impaired memory and organizational skills caused her to misplace things around the house, had forgotten to return her daughter's permission slip on time. Thus, common cognitive problems can interfere with planning and family communication, resulting in frustrating misunderstandings and conflict.

Emotional And Behavioral Symptoms

EMOTIONAL ADJUSTMENT TO MS is an ongoing process that begins at diagnosis and continues over the course of the illness. Considering the unpredictability and potential disability that accompany MS, it is not surprising that depression is very common (see Chapter 2). Untreated depression can have a significant impact on a parent's ability or motivation to carry out the daily activities and responsibilities of parenting. Ms. B, a 30-year-old, single mother with progressive MS, had become socially isolated since having to give up her secretarial job. As she became increasingly depressed, Ms. B relied more and more on her school-aged daughter for companionship, often restricting the child's after-school play time to watching television with her. Her daughter became resentful and emotionally torn, wanting both to spend time with her friends in the neighborhood and to please her mother.

The mood swings, outbursts of temper, and general irritability that sometimes occur with MS can also interfere with parent-child interactions. Children often have particular difficulty understanding a parent's intense and unpredictable emotional state, particularly when they become the easy and available target for these frustrations. When Sarah G came running into the house to ask her father if she could go to the movies with a friend, her father reacted by yelling loudly at her to stop interrupting him. Mr. G's problems with attention, concentration, and memory had been interfering with his efforts to balance his checkbook and pay the monthly bills. When Sarah came into the room, she inadvertently interrupted her father's efforts to concentrate and complete a task that would once have been simple for him. The anger and frustration he felt spilled over to his surprised young daughter, who went back and told her friend she could not go to the movies. This kind of misplaced anger often leaves the parent feeling guilty and the child feeling resentful, hurt, and confused.

Social Consequences

IT IS NOT unusual for a family to renegotiate roles and responsibilities in response to changes in physical or cognitive abilities that result from a chronic illness. Some of the most profound consequences of MS involve the reconfiguration that occurs within the family as its members try to cope with the disease. For example, the breadwinning spouse with MS who becomes unable to continue working may stay at home and take on new parenting responsibilities while the well-spouse returns to the workforce. Other families may find themselves facing the necessity of sharing parenting responsibilities with individuals from outside the family (e.g., home health workers). In its most dramatic form, reconfiguration within the family may involve divorce or separation. Less obvious reconfigurations involve the emotional withdrawal of one or both partners from each other and/or from their parenting roles. Single parents who have MS seem to be particularly at risk for increased role-related stress because they often have no partner with whom they can share financial, household, and parenting responsibilities.

Some parents assume that, because of their MS, they can no longer be as involved in their children's social, recreational, and athletic activities. MS symptoms, transportation problems, and architectural barriers may indeed prevent a parent from participating in the way he or she once did. However, it is important for parents to assess each situation carefully, pursue all their options, and seek assistance before depriving themselves and their children of their participation.

Another common assumption made by parents is that their children will be embarrassed to be seen with a parent who uses a cane or a wheelchair. In fact, the supportive presence of the parent usually outweighs any embarrassment, and many children are proud of parents who have overcome difficulties associated with their MS. Younger children are particularly interested in having their parent come to school to talk to the class about physical disability or give the children a demonstration ride in a wheelchair or scooter. Adolescents (who may be embarrassed by their mothers and fathers whether they have MS or not) often engage their parent's help to write a research paper about MS for one of their classes.

Financial Consequences

A FAMILY S FINANCIAL situation may change considerably as a result of a parent's MS. Such changes can occur for a variety of reasons, including the high cost of medical care, the loss of income that results from the MS-parent's reduced ability to work, or the well-spouse's need to leave work in order to perform additional care giving or parenting functions. Many families are thus left with severely limited financial resources (see Chapter 12).

For some families, especially those that are headed by single parents, this may result in the need to live with extended family under less than ideal circumstances. For others, it means a more gradual change in lifestyle. Individuals who are still physically able to drive may be unable to afford automobile-related expenses. This may leave them with few options for transportation, particularly if they are uncomfortable asking family members and friends for rides. Common family activities such as eating out, gift giving, and summer vacations may all be negatively affected by limited finances.

Thus, family activities may be far more limited by restricted finances than by the parent's disability. Many parents worry that they will no longer be able to provide adequately for their children and that their children, as well as family members and friends, will conclude that they are no longer good parents. Faced with such financial limitations, it is often helpful to involve children in the process of making choices. This conveys the message that although the family can no longer do all of their favorite activities, each family member can help to choose one or two.

Children's Responses to a Parent's Illness

What Does The Research Tell Us?

PARENTS WHO HAVE MS generally agree that their children cope relatively well with the stress of MS in their lives. Indeed, recent studies of families with an MS parent have shown most of the children to be thriving socially, emotionally, and academically. It is clear that a parent's physical illness can potentially serve some positive functions within families, such as bringing family members closer together and helping children learn responsibility and gain independence. Parents often report that their children are more caring and sensitive to the needs of the disabled and that they have a greater sense of responsibility than most children their age.

However, a series of interviews with parents and children showed that the adults tended to underestimate the emotional impact of the MS on their children's lives, whereas the children reported more coping difficulties than their parents described them as having. The children in this study, who ranged in age from 7-18 years, were adapting quite well to their parent's physical limitations. However, they were having much greater difficulty with the parent's mood changes and the emotional climate of anxiety, sadness, and tension within the household. Many of the children felt that they were unfairly targeted by their parent's anger and frustration, and described a "walking on eggshells" atmosphere in the home. Some children hesitated to ask their parent MS-related questions for fear of upsetting the parent even further.

The conclusions reached in this particular study were that the children seemed to be coping more comfortably with the MS than their parents were. Having been reassured that their parent was not going to die and was going to continue to take care of them, these children were making a satisfactory adjustment to the presence of MS in their lives. The parents, however, seemed to be trying to reassure themselves that the MS was not going to have any negative impact on their children's lives. In their need to reassure themselves in this way, many were overlooking some of the MS-related tensions in the household and the effect these tensions were having on the children. For the same reasons, the parents were reluctant to seek professional help with these emotional issues. Rather than seeing family counseling as a valuable tool to cope with the unavoidable stresses imposed by a chronic illness, these parents tended to see counseling either as unnecessary or as an admission of failure in their parenting efforts.

Stressful Events For Children

CERTAIN DISEASE-RELATED EVENTS, such as a parent's hospitalization for an acute exacerbation, cause children to feel more vulnerable and upset. Children experience increased anxiety during these periods of separation from their parent. Hospitals are typically seen by children as places for the very sick or the dying. They may even have had a grandparent who was hospitalized prior to his or her death. Children, particularly those of single parents, may also dislike the prospect of being cared for by someone else while the parent is away. The anticipated and actual disruption of their daily routine as a result of the parent's absence is a major source of anxiety and sometimes resentment.

Depending on the reasons for a hospital admission, the child may also be concerned about the type of treatment the parent is receiving, and how long it will be before the parent is able to return home. During hospitalizations, it is important for parents and children to stay in close contact via telephone, letters, or cards. Visits to the hospital provide children with the opportunity to see for themselves how their parent is doing.

Another event that can be very frightening for children is seeing their parent fall. Children can feel quite helpless in this situation, especially if they are not strong enough to lift the parent up again. One young boy became so concerned about his mother's falls that he never wanted to be at home alone with her. A visiting nurse came to the house to make recommendations to the mother about adaptive equipment for the home and to teach the boy and his mother how to deal with any future falls more comfortably and safely.

How Children Perceive Multiple Sclerosis

IT IS IMPORTANT to remember that a child's developmental level influences what he or she can understand about a parent's illness. For example, young children tend to think in concrete terms and have only a limited understanding of the passage of time. As a result, a young child would be likely to believe that his mother's brace is in place because her leg was broken in a fall she took last week and will come off again as soon as her leg heals. Adolescents are able to think about things in more complex and abstract terms, which enables them to think about different possible outcomes.

In addition to their developmental differences, children often have personal preferences about the kind and amount of information they want about MS, the form in which that information is conveyed, and who should provide the information. Some children may want to read information on their own, asking questions as they come up, whereas others may prefer to accompany their parent to an MS-related appointment where they can direct questions to members of the healthcare team. Older children and adolescents tend to be concerned about getting MS themselves or passing it on to their own children; younger children want to know if people can "catch" MS and if their parent will die.

It is critical to consider how a child's developmental level influences his or her perceptions, interpretations, and responses to a parent's MS. For example, separation anxiety is particularly common in younger children when they begin to attend school. They may worry that something bad will happen to the MS parent while they are gone, or that the parent will need help and will not have anyone to provide it. Children in single-parent families may be at increased risk for anxiety, having already felt the loss of one parent from the home.

Some children who feel torn between being with their parent and attending school may even fake illness in order to stay home and look after their parent. This is more likely to occur when parents look to their children for relief from feelings of fear, helplessness, or loneliness. Children can follow their academic and social routines more comfortably when they are reassured that the parent wants them to pursue these activities, knows how to take care of him- or herself, and has resources to call upon if help is needed. Interestingly, this same issue repeats itself when older children prepare to leave home for college or work. These children need similar reassurances that the parent is proud of their growing independence and can manage comfortably and safely even in their absence.

Children's Responsibilities

IT IS NOT unusual for children who have an ill parent to assume responsibilities beyond their years. Many children who have a parent with MS are assigned more than the usual number of chores around the house. Although some children who have such increased responsibilities may become overly mature or serious for their age, most of them continue to develop and thrive in spite of the added stresses and responsibilities.

More serious problems can result when school age and adolescent children become the sole caregivers for their parents because of too few community services and the unavailability of other adults to provide care. In these situations, the kinds of physical contact that are required for personal care activities (e.g., bathing and bowel and bladder care) often cause significant discomfort for both the child and the parent. In addition to their emotional distress, children who have such responsibilities may be absent from school often enough to interfere with their schoolwork and cause them to miss out on other important age-appropriate activities.

In some families, children may begin to take on so many additional responsibilities that they function as a co-parent for siblings. These added responsibilities may include meal preparation, cleaning, and even disciplining younger children. Although these children may initially enjoy their new-found sense of authority and special position, they are likely to become quite confused about their role in the family, particularly since they still need nurturance and supervision themselves. They are also likely to resent the interference of these extra responsibilities with their own activities.

Although these are fairly typical problems that MS can present for parenting, it is important to recognize that there are marked individual differences in family strengths, coping styles, and social and emotional resources. Some individual and family characteristics seem to be related to better coping and adjustment to MS, including flexible problem-solving skills, a strong social support network, and the willingness to seek and accept help as needed.

Recommendations

Communicating With Children About MS

TALKING OPENLY WITH children about MS helps relieve their anxiety about the parent's health and their own security and well-being. When parents are reluctant to talk about the disease, children often misinterpret silence as an indication that the problem is so terrible that it cannot be discussed. Most children are acutely aware when a parent has a health problem or is not functioning up to par. When no explanation is given, children use their vivid imaginations to conjure up an explanation for themselves, and their guesses are almost always worse than the reality. Most children are relieved to hear the truth.

In addition, some children become quite angry when they find out that others were told this important information before they were. Older children in particular may resent that distant relatives or people outside the family were trusted with this information while they were not.

Keeping secrets takes a lot of energy and diminishes good communication. The longer MS is kept a secret from children, the greater the likelihood is that they will hear this important piece of information from someone outside the family. Parents who can talk directly with their children about MS convey a message of strength and confidence, a message that no matter what the future brings, they will continue to love and care for their children. Furthermore, parents who talk openly with children about the disease and their efforts to cope with it are also laying the groundwork for effective parent-child communications about other family issues. They are letting their children know that families handle problems together and support each other's efforts to cope with whatever comes their way.

When responding to common questions and concerns, it is essential to take into consideration each child's age and developmental level and not to overwhelm them with information they cannot understand. Thus, you might find, at least initially, that talking with each child individually enables you to tailor your discussion to the child's level of understanding. You can also ask children how they would like to learn more about MS—by reading a book with you or alone, watching a video, or accompanying you to the doctor's office. You may even be able to schedule a special appointment just for them to ask the doctor questions. Many age-appropriate educational materials are available through your local chapter of the National MS Society as well as chapter-sponsored meetings designed for children (see Chapter 13).

When talking with your children about MS symptoms, it is often useful to describe and demonstrate the symptoms in a fairly concrete way that they can more easily understand. You might, for instance, describe MS fatigue as the feeling that they would get if they tried to walk around with weights on their arms and legs. Vision problems might be described as feeling like one is looking through a mesh screen all the time or looking at a movie screen with a big hole in the middle. You might convey the feeling of spasticity by letting your child try walking with an elastic bandage wound around each leg. It is important to remember that children will have the greatest difficulty understanding symptoms that they cannot see.

Similarly, it is often useful to let children experiment with assistive devices (e.g., canes, crutches, a motorized scooter, or a wheelchair). They will feel less intimidated by equipment that they have handled and used themselves.

Educational sessions for children, conducted by members of the MS healthcare team, may also be available at MS centers. These meetings provide children with age-appropriate information about the disease, an opportunity to become familiar with the treatment setting and healthcare personnel, and an opportunity to ask questions that they may be hesitant to ask their parents.

In spite of having been told about MS by their parents, some children do not ask many questions or seem very interested in talking about it. It may not be easy to know if your child has concerns about MS because many children keep their worries to themselves. Sometimes children do not know how to ask their questions; sometimes they hesitate to ask questions for fear of upsetting their parents and possibly making the MS worse. Some children who hesitate to talk about their concerns may express them in their behavior. For example, children who are worried about a parent's recent hospitalization or physical worsening may have difficulty sleeping, become very clingy, or complain of physical symptoms in order to stay home from school. Others may act out in school or lose interest in their schoolwork.

Although there is certainly no need to talk incessantly about MS, it is occasionally useful to ask your child if he or she has any questions or concerns. This is particularly important any time there are obvious changes in your situation, such as going into the hospital for treatment, starting to inject yourself with one of the disease-modifying medications, starting to use an ambulatory aid, or thinking about leaving your job. Raising these issues with your children reassures them that they can say what is on their mind and gives them the vocabulary they might need to ask their questions.

Coping With The Physical Consequences Of MS

RELAPSING OR EPISODIC MS, which is characterized by exacerbations or changes over time, may be particularly confusing and stressful for children because of frequent transitions between stable periods, with low level or no symptoms, and periods of symptom flare-up. However, even those parents who have a more steadily progressive course of MS can experience changes in their symptoms from one day to the next. The unpredictability of symptoms from day to day often makes it difficult to plan activities and carry them out in a consistent manner.

Because families must somehow learn to deal with the realities of the illness as they are, the recommended strategy is to try to take each day as it comes. Make plans with your children, explaining that if you are unable to carry out those plans as originally scheduled, you will give them a rain check. Be sure to let them know that you share their disappointment and frustration. In addition, try to give them some explanation of the problem you are having. Although children can understand the concept of "having a bad day," it is probably best to let them know in a straightforward way what is causing you discomfort and interfering with the planned activity.

Enlisting the help of trusted family members and friends to participate in recreational and other physical activities with your children can be very helpful. Although parents often assume that other people are too busy to help, many friends and family say they have wanted to provide assistance in some way but believed their offers of help would be refused or interpreted as intrusive. When asking for help from others, your request is most likely to be fulfilled if you are specific and clear about your needs. You might, for example, ask a close friend or relative to accompany your daughter on a Girl Scout overnight trip or drive your son to his music lesson once a week. Ideally, it is helpful to have several individuals who can provide support to you and your family so that no one person becomes overwhelmed.

If you begin to find yourself depending on your children for help with personal care activities such as getting dressed or going to the bathroom, talk with your doctor, nurse, or other healthcare provider to make sure you have examined and exhausted all other possible resources.

Coping With Cognitive Impairments

IF A PARENT or other family member believes that cognitive symptoms may be present, a neuropsychological evaluation can help identify specific problems as well as areas of strength. This, in turn, will make it possible to identify strategies that parents and children can use to improve their communication and reduce stress (see Chapter 2). For example, if a parent has difficulty with concentration, it is important to reduce distractions when discussing important issues with the children. Such discussions are more likely to be successful when they take place in a quiet environment without a television or radio in the background. Similarly, a mother who has problems with attention and concentration may have difficulty answering a child's homework questions and preparing dinner at the same time. It is important to explain the difficulty to your child and then try to arrange a specific time and place to work on the homework when other distractions are at a minimum.

A family calendar is another useful strategy for minimizing confusion in the household. Each family member's appointments and activities can be posted in a central location to which parents and children have easy access. This makes it easier for a parent who has memory problems to keep track of the family's complicated schedule. Older children can be encouraged to write their commitments on the calendar and to take responsibility for reminding Mom or Dad if they will need a ride.

Coping With Emotional And Behavioral Changes

PARENTS LIVING WITH MS may find themselves experiencing a variety of uncomfortable emotions, either as a reaction to the numerous changes and stresses in their lives or as part of the disease process itself. It is time to talk to your physician or other healthcare provider if you are feeling or acting "not like your old self" or are taking out these uncomfortable feelings on your children or others close to you. Seeking help with emotional changes is similar to seeking help for any of your other MS-related problems. A mental health professional who is knowledgeable about MS can provide you with a better understanding of the emotional changes you are experiencing as well as treatment and management strategies for dealing with them. This, in turn, will make it easier for you to talk with your children about your moods and reassure them that they are not (always) the reason for your frustration or sadness.

Help For Parents And Children

THE PREFERRED APPROACH to dealing with most kinds of family issues is a preventive one, involving education about MS, the promotion of positive mental health, and the development and use of adaptive coping strategies. For families living with chronic illness, periodic meetings with a mental health professional to ask questions, talk about areas of concern and distress, identify family strengths and effective coping strategies, and learn alternative strategies where needed, are highly recommended. This kind of periodic, supportive interaction with a knowledgeable professional can effectively promote family well-being and prevent smaller problems from turning into crises. Then, if individual family members, or the family as a whole, begin to experience significant distress, the family is able to turn to a resource person with whom they are already familiar and comfortable. This professional can help determine if additional services are needed— such as marital counseling, a psychiatric evaluation of a family member's depression, or individual therapy—and make the appropriate referrals.

The goal of supportive, educational interventions with families is to enhance their efforts to cope with the intrusion of MS into their lives. With all psychosocial interventions, professionals need to acknowledge and respect the individuality of families as they work to accommodate the impact of MS on their lives. There is no one plan that works for every family. Each family, with the help and support of the healthcare team, must find its own best way.

Additional Readings

National MS Society Publications
  (available by calling 1-800-FIGHT-MS (1-800-344-4867) or
  online at http://www.nationalmssociety.org/library.asp)
Keep S'myelin—A quarterly newsletter for children ages 6–12 who have
  a parent with MS—available in hard copy or in the Society's
  online library at http://www.nationalmssociety.org/library.asp
O'Connell D. *When a Parent Has MS: A Teenager's Guide Teen InsideMS Online*—
  2002. *Quarterly online magazine (nationalmssociety.org/Teen%20InsideMS.
  asp)*
King M. Someone You Know Has MS: A Book for Families.

General Readings

Kalb R, Miller D. Psychosocial Issues. In: Kalb R, (ed.) *Multiple Sclerosis:
  The Questions You Have; The Answers You Need* (3rd ed.) New York: Demos
  Medical Publishing, 2004.
McCue K. Your kids and your MS. *Inside MS*, 1995;13(2):8.
Portnoy-Worenklein L. What it's really like . . . when mommy is
  seriously ill. *Parents Magazine*, August 2003;78(8):37.
Schwarz SP. Making life easier with kids. *InsideMS*, Fall 1995;13(3):13.
Segal J, Simkins J. *Helping Children with Ill or Disabled Parents*. London and
  Bristol, PA: Jessica Kingsley Publishers, 1996.

7

Parenting a Child with MS

Rosalind Kalb, Ph.D.

Lauren Krupp, M.D.

THE VAST MAJORITY of people with MS are diagnosed between the ages of 20 and 50. We know, however, that kids can get MS too, and that at least some of those people diagnosed as young adults actually had their initial symptoms much earlier. Studies indicate that 2.7-5% of people with MS are diagnosed before the age of 16, and one study identified 49 children below the age of six. The majority of youngsters with MS, however, are between the ages of 10 and 17. This chapter is for mothers and fathers who are facing the added challenges of parenting a child with a chronic, unpredictable illness, particularly one that is generally considered by medical professionals, educators, insurance companies, and the general public to be a disease of adults.

The most important thing for you to know is that you are not alone, and that there are resources available to help you along the way. The National MS Society (USA) and the Multiple Sclerosis Society of Canada have joined in the creation of *Young Persons with MS: A Network for Families with a Child or Teen with MS* (see Recommended Resources). In addition to providing you with the most up-to-date information about MS, the Network can also connect you with other parents, refer you to knowledgeable healthcare professionals, provide assistance with school and social issues, and help you develop plans and strategies for the future. You can contact the Network (in the U.S. by calling 1-866-KIDS W MS or emailing childhoodms@nmss.org, or in Canada by calling 1-866-922-6065) to request copies of *Kids Get MS Too: A Guide for Parents Whose Child or Teen Has MS* and an activity booklet for children entitled *Mighty Special Kids.*

As you read about MS in this book and elsewhere, keep in mind that each person's MS is different; your child's MS will not be exactly like anyone else's. This can be very reassuring for those people whose image of the disease is a severely disabled person with limited options. It can also be frustrating and frightening for those who want and need to know what to expect, what to plan for, and what to do. The fact is that is some people with MS develop one or two symptoms while others develop quite a few. Some become severely disabled, but most do not. Children with MS can grow up to lead full, productive, and enjoyable lives. Your challenge as parents is to learn how to live with the unpredictability of the disease, and to help your child navigate the ordinary milestones of childhood and the teen years, sometimes complicated by the ups and downs of MS. Your goal, as it always has been, will be to help your child become an independent, confident adult—and learning how to manage his or her MS will be an important part of that process.

The Recommended Reading List at the end of the chapter includes sources of general information about MS. You can also contact your local chapter of the National MS Society (800-FIGHT-MS) for additional materials or visit the National MS website at www.nationalmssociety.org. The remainder of this chapter focuses on the areas of major concern for parents who have a child or teen with MS.

What We Know about MS in Children

WHILE A COMPREHENSIVE overview of multiple sclerosis (MS) is beyond the scope of this chapter, there are certain issues relating to the diagnosis and management of the disease in children that are particularly important for parents to know.

Diagnosing MS in Children and Teens

FIRST ARE THE special challenges related to making an MS diagnosis. The accepted criteria for diagnosing MS require that the physician be able to find evidence of at least two separate and distinct neurologic events (attacks), that occurred at least one month apart in different areas of the central nervous system (brain, optic nerves, and spinal cord). In addition, the doctor cannot make the diagnosis without first ruling out all other possible explanations for the attacks and related symptoms.

When the physician sees a youngster who has experienced an episode of neurologic symptoms, he or she must try to determine if these symptoms are a one-time event (referred to as acute disseminated encephalomyelitis—ADEM), which requires no ongoing treatment, or the initial episode of what will subsequently turn out to be MS. If it is MS, the doctor will want to begin treatment as soon as possible. Since ADEM is known to occur in children (most commonly following a viral illness), making the diagnosis can be difficult. The difficulty is compounded by the fact that the symptoms can be similar and some physicians think that symptoms of ADEM can actually recur. More research about ADEM is needed in order to clarify this issue. In the meantime, this means that parents may get different opinions about their child's diagnosis from different doctors, and it may take some time to arrive at a definitive answer.

Making Treatment Decisions

ONCE THE DIAGNOSIS of MS has been established, the doctor will likely recommend treatment with one of the disease-modifying therapies that have been approved by FDA and/or Health Canada. These medications, while not specifically approved for use in children, appear to be safe and well-tolerated in individuals under the age of 18. They are increasingly being prescribed to youngsters with MS based on physicians' shared clinical experience, but opinions among doctors regarding which medication to use vary greatly. Once again, this means that parents might hear very different recommendations from different doctors. Few doctors would disagree with the statement that medicine—and particularly the treatment of MS—is as much art as science, and this is particularly true in the treatment of children with MS. Your child's healthcare team will work with you and your child to identify the best treatment options, given your child's particular history and symptoms, and make changes as necessary as time goes on.

Unfortunately, the primary treatment options at this time are all long-term, injectable medications. Receiving or giving oneself the injections on a regular basis is challenging for anyone—adult or child—particularly since these medications do not relieve symptoms or make a person feel better. The injectables are designed to reduce the number and severity of attacks, and slow disease progression, and must therefore be used on a consistent basis, regardless of how the person is feeling at the time. Parents often find it difficult to explain to children and teens why it is essential to take a medication that causes discomfort going in and does not make a person feel better once it is there. And, long-term therapy is a very difficult concept for youngsters to understand, since they are more used to taking a medication (e.g., an antibiotic for strep throat or an ear infection), that solves the problem after several days (and may even taste good).

Dealing with a Relapsing-Remitting Disease

THE VAST MAJORITY of people with MS begin with a relapsing-remitting course. This means that the person experiences acute, time-limited attacks (also called relapses, exacerbations, flare-ups), which are defined as the appearance of new symptoms or the worsening of existing symptoms, lasting at least 24 hours. To be a true attack, the episode must also be separated from the prior attack by at least one month. The attacks (which may or may not be treated with a short course of high-dose corticosteroids) are generally associated with inflammation in the brain or spinal cord. Once the attack subsides, the symptoms may disappear entirely, or the person may be left with some residual problems. During the time between attacks, however, the MS is stable, with no evidence of progression.

Although the attacks of MS come and go, the disease-modifying treatments need to continue without interruption in order to be effective. This can pose a significant challenge for parents and children. No child likes to take medication when he or she is feeling fine (e.g., between attacks). During these periods of remission, particularly if all the symptoms have subsided, it is virtually impossible for youngsters (and often their parents) to believe that the MS is still invisibly active inside the body. Everyone wants to get on with normal life, forgetting about the disease for a while—even believing that it has disappeared once and for all; regular injections are an uncomfortable reminder. Since remissions can last for months, helping children understand why they need to continue taking their injections can be quite difficult. Parents and healthcare providers need to work together to support adherence to the treatment plan.

Recognizing a Pseudoexacerbation

WHEN PEOPLE WITH MS become overly tired, or their bodies become overheated by exercise or a fever (caused, for example, by a viral or bacterial infection), they may experience what are called pseudoexacerbations. The episodes can feel like true attacks of MS because old symptoms may become more active—such as blurry vision or increased feelings of numbness or pins-and-needles. Or a new symptom may briefly rear its head. Unlike a true exacerbation, however, these symptoms disappear as soon as the body cools down again, usually lasting no more than an hour or two following intense exercise, or as long as the fever remains elevated. These brief changes are thought to occur because an elevation in core body temperature interferes with nerve conduction, which disrupts the transfer of messages within the central nervous system that controls the body's normal feelings and functions. It is important for parents and children to realize that these pseudoexacerbations are not dangerous, and do not represent a change or increase in underlying disease activity. They are simply the body's way of announcing that it is overheated. Children who feel well enough to be active, participate in sports or other hobbies, and keep up with their friends, need to be encouraged to do so. Their bodies will tell them if they need to slow down for a little while. They can also learn various cooling strategies to use during sports activities or when the weather is very hot.

Dealing with Progressive Disease

IN THE ABSENCE of treatment, most people with MS are likely at some point to transition from a relapsing-remitting disease course to secondary-progressive (SP) MS. SPMS is generally characterized by steadier disease progression, with or without exacerbations. This progression can be relatively slow and uneventful for some, and more problematic for others. The hope among MS experts is that the injectable, disease-modifying medications will help to delay this transition and/or reduce its impact. If at any point the physician decides that the injectable medication your child is taking no longer seems to be effective in managing the disease or slowing progression, there are other medications that can be prescribed. You can read about the various medications commonly used in MS on the National MS Society website at www.nationalmssociety.org/treatments.asp.

Managing the Symptoms

ONE OF THE challenges of living with MS is that the symptoms it can cause are so varied—and so variable from one person to another. MS can cause fatigue, vision changes, stiffness, weakness, sensory problems such as numbness and tingling or pain, tremor, imbalance, changes in bladder or bowel function, changes in sexual function, emotional changes including mood swings and depression, and problems with thinking and memory. Fortunately, most people do not experience all of these symptoms, and some may experience only a few of them. While no parent likes to think of a child having to deal with any of these problems, the good news is that there are a variety of strategies for managing them.

Recognizing What's MS and What's Not

THE LIST OF possible symptoms is so long that it is sometimes hard to figure out what is caused by MS and what is not. Having MS does not protect a child from the regular illnesses and injuries of childhood, and your child will look to you to help sort out what's what. Knowing the symptoms that MS can cause will help prepare you; your child's healthcare provider will want to know about any new symptoms, or changes in old symptoms, that last longer than a day or so.

For a detailed description of the various symptoms that can occur, you can consult one of the general books about MS listed at the end of the chapter. Or, you can read about them on the National MS Society website (www.nationalmssociety.org/symp-toms.asp.

Visible and Invisible Symptoms

THE PHYSICAL SYMPTOMS of MS tend to be fairly easy to spot; a child who is experiencing pain or weakness or stiffness is likely to be able to describe it. The less visible a symptom is, the harder it may be for you to recognize or understand. The most common of these is fatigue. While fatigue in MS can result from a multitude of factors, including some medications and/or sleep disturbances caused by physical discomfort or urinary problems, the primary fatigue of MS—sometimes caused lassitude—is caused directly by the disease itself. This fatigue can be overwhelming at times, and may not be relieved by rest or sleep. Fortunately, there are activities as well as medications that have been found to be helpful in managing this type of fatigue. Aerobic exercise and the use of appropriate mobility devices to conserve energy can be very helpful.

A child complaining of this type of fatigue is not being lazy or avoiding chores; MS fatigue is reported by many adults with MS to be their most debilitating symptom. It makes it very difficult for many adults to function in the workplace, and may interfere with your child's ability to participate fully at school, even if he or she has no visible physical symptoms. There are effective strategies for coping with MS-related fatigue; adjusting one's schedule, for example, so that the most demanding activities are done in the morning (when fatigue is typically less) is one of many that can be used to combat this symptom. Your physician or healthcare provider will be able to suggest additional strategies for dealing with MS fatigue.

Cognitive and emotional changes can also be difficult for children, as well as their parents and teachers, to recognize and understand. Cognitive changes are relatively common in MS. While there is some disagreement among clinicians about whether cognitive symptoms are more or less common in children than they are in adults, experience suggests that they can occur in childhood MS as well as in adults with the disease. Studies indicate that approximately 50% of people with MS will experience some changes in their cognitive functions over the course of the disease, with the most commonly reported problems being with learning and memory, the processing of incoming information (attention and concentration), planning and decision-making, processing visual information, and understanding and using language. It is important to be aware of the possibility of these types of problems because they can occur at any point in the disease, even as an initial symptom. That means that cognitive and emotional changes can occur in a child who has a lot of physical changes or someone who has none.

These usually subtle changes can interfere with school performance. Some MS experts recommend that children have regular cognitive evaluations beginning at the time of diagnosis, in order to establish the child's baseline abilities and detect any problems that may crop up along the way. Early recognition of a child's problems with thinking or memory makes it possible for the school to address any special needs a child might have in the classroom. Special accommodations, such as sitting at the front of the classroom for example, can help overcome limitations in attention that some children with MS may experience. A child with MS who is experiencing academic difficulties may benefit from an evaluation by a psychologist or neuropsychologist who can make the appropriate recommendations to the school for improving learning and attention.

Navigating the Healthcare System

ONE OF THE biggest challenges parents face is finding and accessing the best possible care for their child. MS is a relatively uncommon illness (approximately 400,000 people in the United States, compared to 9.6 million with cancer, for example, or 15,000,000 with diabetes) and MS in children is actually relatively rare. As a result, many—if not most—physicians and other health professionals, hospitals, and insurance companies may have no experience with youngsters with MS, and may not even know that early-onset MS is possible. This means that at the same time you are educating yourself about MS, you are probably going to have to educate others as well. You will likely need to advocate for your child every step of the way. Arming yourself with information about the disease and available resources will be your very best strategy in this advocacy effort.

Finding the Right Doctor for Your Child

CHILDREN WITH MS are being cared for by a variety of physicians, including family practitioners, pediatricians, adult neurologists (both general neurologists and MS specialist neurologists), and pediatric neurologists. Your National MS Society chapter will be able to give you the names of any physicians in the area who have an interest and expertise in treating children. Given, however, that most physicians have little or no experience with MS in youngsters, there may not be anyone close to you who has ever seen a child or teen with MS. If there are none within a reasonable distance, you have a couple of other options. You can travel to a pediatric MS Center (see Recommended Resources) or your local physician can consult with the neurologists at these centers or with the Society's Professional Resource Center (by calling 1-866-MS-TREAT or by emailing MD_info@nmss.org). Of the few experts focusing on childhood MS, most are eager to offer suggestions and support to local doctors. Whichever option(s) you choose, it is important that both you and your child feel comfortable with the doctor and his or her staff, able to communicate your questions and concerns, and supported in your efforts to manage the disease. You also need to feel confident that the health-care team is a partner in your advocacy efforts with insurance companies and the school system. Particularly in a disease for which there are no sure-fire answers, the relationship with the doctor is a critical component of the coping and adaptation process.

Encouraging Your Child's Relationship with the Doctor

As is true of medicine in general, but particularly with a chronic disease in which there are very few clear-cut answers, the person's relationship with the physician and other clinicians (e.g., the nurse, physical therapist, occupational therapist, counselor, etc.) is an integral part of the treatment. Ideally, the patient is the hub of the treatment team, whether the team is located in one comprehensive care facility or is spread out in many different offices. The patient's needs determine the treatment(s), and his or her responses to the care provide the feedback that is so essential to clinicians' treatment decisions. Over the course of the disease, your child will learn to partner with the healthcare team in his or her own care.

With very young children, the parent obviously acts as the child's surrogate—providing information to the doctor and explanations to the child, answering questions, making decisions. While it is often a parent's instinct to shield a child from something that may be frightening, withholding information—such as the name of the disease—is not beneficial. Even school-age children need to be part of the communication process since this is the way that they will begin to develop their own relationship and partnership with the healthcare team.

By the time a child is in high school, he or she may well want some time alone with the doctor or nurse. Parents can encourage this by coming to an agreement with their child and the doctor that recognizes the child's need for privacy but also makes clear that important decisions need to rest with the parents. As in virtually all areas of development, the teen years are a time of preparation for independence and self-reliance, and the MS arena is no different. The goal is to help kids become ready to manage their own MS, work effectively with their doctors and other providers, and make healthy decisions and choices on their own behalf. This is a gradual process that begins with helping your child develop a comfortable relationship with his or her doctor. By the late teen years, your child will need to be making many of his or her own treatment decisions. While this can be difficult for parents to handle, it is just one more part of your teenager's need to forge an independent road. Like many other areas of life, it means that your child may sometimes make decisions that you would make differently for him or her, or for yourself. Your best strategy is to try and ensure that your child maintains a good relationship with his or her doctor and access to accurate, up-to-date information, and then be available to offer guidance and support when the need arises.

While parents generally see their children off into the world with a sigh of relief, a pang (or more) of anxiety, and a wave of sadness, parents of a child with MS face an even greater challenge. You will want more than anything to be able to watch over your youngster, make sure he or she is eating right, getting enough rest, taking medications on a consistent basis, and doing whatever else the doctor has recommended. As with all the other health and wellness issues that worry parents of teens and young adults these days, however, the choices will ultimately be your child's to make. While always important, your child's relationship with the healthcare team can be vital at this time. Many kids who resist listening to or confiding in their parents at this time will stay in close touch with their doctors.

Dealing with Insurance Issues

SINCE INSURANCE PROGRAMS vary so widely from one country to another, and one insurance company to another, this section provides only general recommendations. More detailed information is available in Chapter 10 of this book and in the American and Canadian versions of *Kids Get MS Too: A Guide for Parents Whose Child or Teen Has MS* (see Recommended Resources and Additional Readings at the end of the chapter). The most important thing to keep in mind is that getting and maintaining health insurance for your child is a critical step in obtaining the care he or she will need along the way. There are a variety of resources available to help you navigate the challenges relating to insurance, including your state's insurance commissioner's office (http://www.patientrights.com/links/links7.htm) and the National MS Society. The Society chapter closest to you (call 1-800-FIGHT-MS) can help you find answers to your insurance questions, and Georgetown University maintains a website that describes health insurance options in each state (www.healthinsuranceinfo.net).

In the meantime, familiarize yourself with the coverage offered by your current policy. You will be in a far better position to advocate for your child if you have spent time getting to know the basic elements of your plan, including:

▶ Eligibility requirements (who is covered under what circumstances).
▶ Benefits (which services/treatments are specifically included or excluded and what are the limits on the coverage provided).
▶ Regulatory information (who is responsible for enforcing the provisions of the plan, and to whom would appeals be addressed if needed).
▶ Coverage parameters affecting cost (how can you utilize your plan most effectively to minimize out-of-pocket costs).
▶ Grievance procedures (what is the grievance/appeal process).

Navigating the Education System

VIRTUALLY EVERY PARENT of a child diagnosed with MS has concerns about the impact of the disease on the child's education. The concerns are *immediate*—What if my child misses too many days of school? What if my child cannot participate in classroom or extracurricular activities? What if my child can't do the required work? Can my child's school provide what he or she needs? How will teachers and classmates respond to my child's MS? And the concerns are *long-range*—Will my child be able to graduate with his or her peers? Will my child be able to go to college? Will my child be able to succeed?

There are two important things to keep in mind. First, the healthcare team will help you and your child learn how best to manage the symptoms of MS, and how to identify and implement effective accommodations in the school setting. Second, there are laws governing the rights of children in different educational settings at different levels. Specific educational issues are addressed in the American and Canadian versions of *Kids Get MS Too: A Guide for Parents Whose Child or Teen Has MS*. The National MS Society and the Canadian MS Society can refer you to appropriate resources in your area.

Managing Your Own Feelings

PARENTING IS NEVER easy. Given the complexities of MS and its treatment, you may find yourself struggling more than usual to figure out how best to help your child. The first step in taking care of your child is taking care of yourself. Just as the flight attendant instructs you to put on your own oxygen mask before helping anyone with you who requires assistance, your ability to support your child's adaptation to MS will depend on your own level of health and well-being. Dealing with your feelings about this unexpected diagnosis is a good place to start. Common feelings among parents who have a child with MS include anxiety, grief, anger, and even guilt. The *guilt* is most often related to parents' concerns that they might have caused the disease to happen, or somehow failed to keep it from happening. While there is much that is still unknown about MS, we do know that there is nothing that you or your child did to make this happen. MS is thought to be an immune-mediated disease that is triggered by some viral or bacterial agent in the environment, in people who have a genetic predisposition to respond to it. The risk of developing MS in the general population is about 1 in 750. The level of risk rises—to approximately 1 in 40—for any individual who has a close relative with the disease, and is higher still in families in which several people have MS.

The *sadness* is related primarily to feelings of loss. Every parent wants his or her children to be healthy and happy, and every parent works hard to make it so. No one wants a child to have to live with a chronic illness, deal with uncomfortable symptoms, cope with impairments of any kind, or be limited in the things he or she can do or enjoy. Parents are saddened by their inability to prevent these things from happening, and find it difficult to watch their children having to deal with these issues. The good news is that the medical community has learned a great deal over the past 10-15 years about how to manage the disease and reduce its impact on everyday life.

The unpredictability of MS makes parents feel *anxious* and *angry* as well. Moms and dads want to know what is going to happen next, and what is going to happen in the future, and they may feel very frustrated when no one can give them answers. The normal questions that all parents have—will my child have a good life ... get a good education ... find a good job ... get married ... have children ... be happy ... be healthy ... are magnified when a child has MS. Anxiety and anger are also normal responses to feeling out of control, and unpredictability and unanswered questions always make people feel less in control. Because of the unpredictability of MS, the lack of clarity concerning the diagnosis, and the limited numbers of children with this disease on which to base predictions and recommendations, parents do not have a clear road map to tell them what to do.

The best way to deal with these kinds of uncomfortable feelings is to recognize what they are and where they come from, and develop coping strategies that feel right for you. The first step is to find healthcare providers with whom you and your child feel comfortable and confident. While no one has all the answers, you will find that being able to communicate openly about the diagnostic issues and the treatment options will go a long way toward helping you feel a bit more in control of the situation. As your youngster grows and approaches different developmental milestones (e.g., entering the teenage years, preparing to leave home, etc.), the healthcare team will be able to help you and your child make the necessary transitions.

Some people also need to find others with whom to discuss their feelings—a close friend, a National MS Society staff member, a support group, or a counselor; others find that exercise or meditation or an engaging hobby help them maintain a sense of balance and reduce the stress. The particular method you choose does not matter; what matters is that you take care of your own emotional needs so that you are better able to help your child and engage in the kind of creative problem-solving that is likely to be required along the way. If you and your spouse or partner are having difficulty communicating about your respective feelings, or find that your coping strategies differ to the extent that it causes conflict, a family counselor who is familiar with MS can be a helpful resource. You can ask your chapter of the National MS Society for a list of therapists in your area who are familiar with MS.

Parenting Tips Along the Way

WHILE MS IS only one part of your life with your child, it obviously adds some additional complexities to the parent-child relationship. In this section, some of the major concerns that parents have raised about how to help their child along the way are addressed.

Talking about the Diagnosis

PARENTS OFTEN WONDER how much information about MS they should share with their child. No parents want to make their children anxious or sad, and no parents wants to see their children having to deal with life's tougher realities any sooner than necessary. The fact is, however, that children know when they do not feel well and they know when their parents are worried or upset. If they sense that something is different or awry, their imaginations will quickly fill in the blanks—typically with something even more frightening than whatever the reality actually is. Your best strategy is to begin sharing age-appropriate information (including the name of the disease) with your child from the beginning. Without this information, it will be much more difficult—and stressful—for your child as he or she undergoes neurologic exams, tests, and treatments. Obviously, five-year-olds do not need or understand as many of the details as teenagers do, and their style of listening, learning, and questioning will be quite different, but the sharing of information can help any child feel more comfortable with the diagnosis and treatment process. There are other benefits as well to this kind of openness:

▶ When children have a better understanding of what is going on, they feel less like victims and more like active participants. Rather than things being done "to them," they feel safer and more involved in the process of dealing with the MS.

▶ Honesty and open communication promote feelings of trust and confidence among family members. They set the stage for shared problem-solving and mutual support in the future, and eliminate the need for secrets relating to MS or any other issues that may come along.

▶ Children gain a feeling of security when they sense that their parents are being open and honest. When parents come across as secretive, unwilling to share information, or afraid to discuss certain topics, children quickly assume that the truth is too awful to deal with, too frightening to handle.

▶ Talking openly with children about MS gives them "permission" to ask their questions and share their feelings and concerns. It also gives them the vocabulary they need to put them into words.

If you are feeling uncertain about how to proceed—and most parents do—the healthcare team, the Family Network, and/or a family counselor can help you figure out age-appropriate ways to begin the discussions with your child.

Helping Your Child Be a "Normal Kid"

MOST PARENTS EXPRESS concerns about how protective to be of a child diagnosed with MS. Their instincts range from wanting to keep their child in a kind of protective cocoon in hopes of preventing anything bad from happening, to wanting to make sure that their child gets to do absolutely everything that all the other kids are doing. The most realistic strategy is somewhere in between. Your son or daughter's physician will let you know if there are any restrictions on your child's activities; your best guidance on a day-to-day basis, however, is likely to come from your child. His or her body will give pretty clear signals. If fatigue is a prominent symptom—as it is for many people with MS—your child will simply not feel up to being very active some days. On the other hand, many children with MS are active in both sports and other extracurricular school activities.

During acute attacks of the disease, fatigue or other symptoms may prevent your child from engaging in physical activities, socializing busily with friends, or even making it to school. During periods of remission, however, both you and your child may feel that everything is back to "normal," with no holds barred. The challenge will be in encouraging your child to listen to his or her body, to avoid becoming overly exhausted, and to learn how to balance periods of activity with rest breaks when needed. Nobody is going to be an instant expert at this—it will be a learning process for your child over the course of the illness. The main thing to keep in mind is that nothing your child does is going to make the MS either better or worse in the long term. The goal is for your son or daughter to be as active and involved as possible, while maintaining an optimal comfort level.

Meeting the Needs of Other Children in the Family

WHENEVER ONE PERSON in a family becomes ill, there is a tendency for everyone's attention and emotional energy to focus—at least for a time—on that person. This is particularly true when the family member is a child. Parents can easily become consumed with worry and with care giving, whether it is hands-on care, trips to doctors, meetings with the school, or telephone calls to insurance companies. This level of focused attention on one family member is acceptable during an acute crisis because everyone in the family expects the crisis to pass. When the illness is chronic, however, the challenge lies in finding ways to deal with the needs of the person who is ill or disabled, while still having enough time, emotions, and energy to ensure the well-being of others in the family as well (see Chapter 2).

When one child in a family is diagnosed with MS, the other children in the family may have a variety of special concerns:

- ▶ Why did this happen—is it my fault?
- ▶ Is my brother/sister going to die?
- ▶ Is it going to happen to me—will I catch it?
- ▶ How come no one is paying attention to me—don't I count anymore?
- ▶ Do I need to get sick so they'll love me too?
- ▶ Would they still love me if they knew how angry I am that he/she got MS?
- ▶ Am I going to be stuck with all the chores around here forever?

As extreme as some of these concerns may sound, they are real and painful—and so uncomfortable that your other children may never say them out loud. It is safe to assume that whenever there is an upset in the family's equilibrium, or a change in the routines of daily life, children will have feelings about it. Your best strategy is to touch base with your other kids as often as you are able, keeping them informed (at an age-appropriate level), asking if they have any questions or worries, and letting them know that you are aware how upsetting some of this must be for them. If at all possible, try to arrange some special alone time with each child—a very little bit can go a very long way. It is also helpful to alert young children's teachers about any disruptions or changes that are going on at home so that the teachers can be on the lookout for behavior changes or emotional distress.

When Your Child's MS Feels Like a Full-Time Job

THIS CHAPTER ENDS with a reminder—*In order to provide the best possible care for your child, you need to make sure that you are tending to your own needs as well.* Just because you have a child with MS does not mean that the other demands in your life will cease; once the initial crisis of the diagnosis or the initial attack has passed, your other children, your spouse, your friends, your colleagues at work, and your boss will gradually expect things to get back to "normal." You may find yourself pulled in countless different directions, with little or no time or energy left for yourself. Because your own health and well-being are so important, not only to you but to those around you, now is the time to develop your support network, learn which stress management strategies work best for you, make sure you are getting enough rest, and carve out at least a little bit of time each day that is just for you. Reach out to the Network for Families—you and your family do not need to be alone.

RECOMMENDED READINGS

Kalb R, (ed.) Multiple Sclerosis: The Questions You Have; The Answers You Need (3rd ed.) New York: Demos Medical Publishing, 2004.

Northrop D, Cooper S. Health Insurance Resource Manual: Options for People with a Chronic Disease or Disability. New York: Demos Medical Publishing, 2003.

Russell LM, Grant AE, Joseph SM, Fee RW. Planning for the Future: Providing a Meaningful Life for a Child with a Disability After Your Death (2nd ed.) Evanston, IL: American Publishing, 1993.

RECOMMENDED RESOURCES (Adapted with permission from *Kids Get MS Too: A Guide for Parents Whose Child or Teen Has MS*, available from the National MS Society and the Multiple Sclerosis Society of Canada).

GENERAL RESOURCES
INFORMATION ON MULTIPLE SCLEROSIS

National Multiple Sclerosis Society www.nationalmssociety.org
Multiple Sclerosis Society of Canada www.mssociety.ca

PHARMACEUTICAL COMPANIES

(*Though these drugs are not approved for use in children, they are, as is mentioned in the text, frequently prescribed for children.*)
Biogen Inc. – MS Active Source℠ (Avonex®)
    www.msactivesource.com
    800-456-2255
Teva Neuroscience – Shared Solutions™ (Copaxone®)

www.sharedsolutions.com

1-800-887-8100

Berlex Laboratories – MS Pathways^{SM} (Betaseron®)

www.mspathways.com

1-800-788-1467

Serono, Inc. – MS Lifelines™ (Rebif®)

www.mslifelines.com

1-877-447-3243

RESOURCES IN THE UNITED STATES
FEDERAL GOVERNMENT

US Department of Health & Human Services

http://www.hhs.gov/

Office of Special Education and Rehabilitation Services (OSERS)

http://www.ed.gov/about/offices/list/osers/nidrr/index.
html?scr=mr

CHILDREN WITH DISABILITIES/CHRONIC ILLNESS

Institute of Disability, University of Minnesota: Division of General
Pediatric and Adolescent Health

http://www.peds.umn.edu/peds-adol/ihd.html

Family Village , Waisman Center, University of Wisconsin-Madison

http://www.familyvillage.wisc.edu/

American Council on Education

http://www.acenet.edu/

Band-Aides and Blackboards

http://www.faculty.fairfield.edu/fleitas/contents.html

IRSC – Internet Resources for Special Children

http://www.irsc.org/

EDUCATION

Office of Special Education Programs at the U.S. Department of
Education

OSEP funds a large information dissemination and technical
assistance network plus there is a customer service specialist for
each state. www.ed.gov/about/offices/osers/osep/index.html
202-205-5507

Office for Civil Rights at the U.S. Department of Education
Technical assistance, pamphlets, complaint information on
Section 504 of the Rehabilitation Act.
www.ed.gov/about/offices/list/ocr/index.html
800-421-3481 voice
877-521-2172 TTY

U.S. Department of Justice
Technical assistance, publications, complaint information on
Titles II and III of the ADA.
www.ada.gov
800-514-0301 voice
800-514-0383 TTY

ADA and IT Technical Assistance Centers
Technical assistance and publications on all aspects of the ADA
and accessible information technology in educational settings.
www.adata.org
800-949-4232 voice/TTY

Parent Training and Information Centers and Community Parent
Resource Centers
Parent centers in each state provide training and information to
help parents participate more effectively with professionals in
meeting the educational needs of children with disabilities.
www.taalliance.org/PTIs.htm
888-248-0822 voice/TTY

EDLAW, Inc.
Maintains a web-based list of attorneys who represent parents
of children with disabilities.
www.edlaw.net/service/attylist.html

National Center on Secondary Education and Transition
NCSET coordinates national resources, offers technical
assistance, and dissiminates information related to secondary
education and transition for youth with disabilities.
http://www.ncset.org

National Dissemination Center for Children and Youth with
Disabilities (NICHCY)
Provides technical assistance and publications on disability
issues—focus is children and youth (birth to age 22) and IDEA.
www.nichcy.org

800-695-0285 · voice/tty
Association on Higher Education and Disability (AHEAD)
Publications, information, and training on higher education
and students with disabilities.
www.ahead.org
781-788-0003 voice/TTY?
781-788-0033 fax

INSURANCE

Covering Kids and Families
www.coveringkidsandfamilies.org
1-877-543-7669
Georgetown University: Health insurance options for each state.
www.healthinsuranceinfo.net.
Medical Information Bureau (MIB)
www.mib.com
617-426-3660 781-751-6130?

RESOURCES IN CANADA
FEDERAL GOVERNMENT

Health Canada http://www.hc-sc.gc.ca/

DISABILITY RESOURCES

Disability WebLinks
http://www.disabilityweblinks.ca/pls/dwl/dl.home
Councils of Ministers of Education, Canada
http://www.cmec.ca/index.en.html

CHILDREN WITH DISABILITIES/CHRONIC ILLNESS

Canadian Association of Family Resource Programs
http://www.frp.ca/
Canadian Coalition for the Rights of Children
http://www.rightsofchildren.ca/
Canadian Institute of Child Health http://www.cich.ca/
Canadian Mental Health Association http://www.cmha.ca/
Family Service Canada http://www.familyservicecanada.org
Hospital for Sick Children http://www.sickkids.on.ca/

Canadian Ministries of Education

In Canada, education is the responsibility of each province and territory. Each provincial ministry of education has been listed below, including contact information. Information regarding special education, or special assistance within the classroom, or otherwise should be available through your child's school; however, as an extra resource, each is listed for your convenience.

Council of Ministers of Education, Canada

95 St. Clair Avenue West, Suite 1106 Toronto, Ontario M4V 1N6
Telephone: (416) 962-8100
Fax: (416) 962-2800
E-mail: cmec@cmec.ca
Website: http://www.cmec.ca/

Alberta Learning

7th Floor, Commerce Place
10155–102 Street
Edmonton, Alberta T5J 4L5
Tel: (780) 427-7219
For toll-free access within Alberta, first dial 310-0000
Fax: (780) 422-1263
E-mail: comm.contact@learning.gov.ab.ca
Web site: http://www.learning.gov.ab.ca/

British Columbia Ministry of Education

Ministry of Education
PO Box 9150, Stn Prov Govt
Victoria BC V8W 9H1
Tel: (250) 356-2500
Fax: (250) 356-5945
Website: http://www.gov.bc.ca/bced/

Manitoba Education, Citizenship and Youth Advanced Education and Training

206-1181 Portage Avenue
Winnipeg, Manitoba R3G 0T3
Phone: (204) 945-7912
Fax: (204) 945-7914
Website: http://www.edu.gov.mb.ca/

New Brunswick Department of Education
　　Place 2000
　　P.O. Box 6000
　　Fredericton, NB E3B 5H1
　　Tel: (506) 453-3678
　　Fax: (506) 453-3325
　　Website: http://www.gnb.ca/0000/

Newfoundland and Labrador Department of Education
　　P.O. Box 8700
　　St. John's, NL A1B 4J6
　　Tel: (709) 729-5097
　　Fax: (709) 729-5896
　　Website: www.gov.nl.ca/edu/
　　Student Support Services:
　　http://www.gov.nf.ca/edu/dept/sss.htm

Northwest Territories Department of Education
　　NWT Education, Culture and Employment
　　Box 1320
　　Yellowknife, NT X1A 2L9
　　OR
　　Early Childhood Education & School Services
　　3rd Floor, Lahm Ridge Towers
　　Yellowknife, NT X1A 2L9
　　Tel: (867) 920-3416
　　Fax: (867) 873-0109

Nova Scotia Department of Education
　　P.O. Box 578
　　2021 Brunswick Street, Suite 402
　　Halifax, Nova Scotia B3J 2S9
　　Tel: (902) 424-5168
　　Fax: (902) 424-0511
　　Website: http://www.ednet.ns.ca/

Ontario Ministry of Education
　　Mowat Block, 900 Bay Street
　　Toronto, Ontario M7A 1L2
　　Tel: (416) 325-2929 or 1-800-387-5514
　　Fax: (416) 325-6348
　　e-mail: info@edu.gov.on.ca

Website: http://www.edu.gov.on.ca/eng/welcome.html

Prince Edward Island Department of Education

Second Floor, Sullivan Building

16 Fitzroy Street

P.O. Box 2000

Charlottetown, PEI C1A 7N8

Tel: (902) 368-4600

Fax: (902) 368-4663

Website: http://www.edu.pe.ca/

Quebec Ministry of Education

1035, rue De La Chevrotière, 16e étage

Québec (Québec) G1R 5A5

Tel: (418) 644-0664

Fax: (418) 646-7551

Website: http://www.meq.gouv.qc.ca/GR-PUB/m_englis.htm

Saskatchewan Education

c/o Special Education Unit

2nd Floor

2220 College Avenue

Regina, Saskatchewan S4P 3V7

Tel: (306) 787-1183

Fax: (306) 787-0277

http://www.sasked.gov.sk.ca/

Yukon Department of Education

Special Programs

Department of Education

Government of Yukon

Box 2703

Whitehorse, Yukon Y1A 2C6

Tel: (867) 667-8000

Toll free (In Yukon) 1-800-661-0408 (local 8000)

Fax: (867) 393-6423

E-mail: shirley.loo@gov.yk.ca

Website:

www.gov.yk.ca/services/departments/special_ed.html

8

Adults with MS and Their Parents

Rosalind Kalb, Ph.D.
Faith Seidman, CSW

M OST CHILDREN AND their parents look forward to the day when the children will be on their own. In our society, one of the major functions of the family is to prepare children to be responsible, independent, and self-supporting members of the community. With the passage of time, the general expectation is that children will become heads of their own households, returning to the parental home for visits, celebrations, reunions, and eventually to provide help or care when their parents become elderly or ill.

Chronic illness and disability can interfere with these expectations. Progressive multiple sclerosis (MS) that is diagnosed during the teens or twenties might interfere with a child's ability to leave home. Some young or middle-aged adults whose MS becomes disabling may find themselves needing parental help or support, and those who are most severely impaired may even return to the parental home because they can no longer afford or manage a place of their own. Because such a reversal of traditional roles and disruption of expected patterns is generally not anticipated, it is important to recognize the complex array of feelings—both positive and negative—that can arise in family members.

On the positive side, there is nothing more reassuring for an adult child with MS than to know that he or she is not alone. The comfort of having parents to turn to for assistance and emotional support is immeasurable. For parents, there can be joy and satisfaction—even a renewed sense of mission—in helping their children to remain as healthy, comfortable, and independent as they can possibly be.

Such a disruption can also create a variety of stresses for the entire family. This chapter describes some of the ways in which family members may react, and discusses possible strategies for coping with these unanticipated events.

Reactions of Adult Children with MS

GIVEN THAT THE expectation of most children growing up in our society is to become independent, the foremost reaction of disabled young adults is often an acute sense of loss over their own destinies. The onset of illness or disability can shatter the feelings of power and invulnerability that propel young people out into the world. When young adults are unable to move out of their parents' home, their dreams are threatened, and they worry that they will never be able to experience the freedom and autonomy that usually come with adulthood.

Older adults who find themselves needing parental care or support after they have already been on their own for a while have an even more complicated adjustment to make. In addition to feeling a loss of control over their own lives, they may also experience a threat to the adult status that they worked so hard to reach and maintain. Those who have been self-supporting and self-directed for a number of years may find that returning to the care and/or support of their parents feels like a giant step backward, not only because their status as adults feels threatened, but also because of the loss of autonomy and privacy. Once one's parents have been asked for help, support (financial or otherwise), or advice, they may tend to slip back into their earlier parental patterns of wanting to guide, protect, or even control. This may be particularly true for the adult child who needs to move back into the parental home; the parents may revert to attitudes or behaviors that were well suited to their child's teenage years, but feel overly intrusive or controlling for an adult who has long been independent. Accustomed to being able to come and go as they please, adult children may find themselves once again needing to live within their parents' schedules and abide by their rules. The parent-child struggles of the past emerge again.

Even for adult children who maintain homes and families of their own, the need for parental help or support can sometimes cause tensions between and within the generations. It may be very difficult for parents and adult children to establish comfortable boundaries. A child may want his or her parents to provide help or advice when they are asked, but feel resentful of unsolicited advice or suggestions; parents who are concerned for their child's welfare may find it difficult to keep their opinions to themselves. Some parents, for example, may feel anxious about a son- or daughter-in-law's willingness or ability to provide sufficient care and emotional or financial support. This may lead the parents to become freer with their advice and opinions than they might otherwise have been, with the result that the son- or daughter-in-law feels pressured or inadequate. Marital tensions are not uncommon in this kind of situation. These types of tensions may be further complicated by disagreements over the care of grandchildren. Grandparents who are called upon to help with certain of the grandchildren's needs may begin to try to control various aspects of their upbringing. This can cause the adult child with MS (and his or her spouse) to feel challenged or inadequate in his or her parenting efforts and resentful of the grandparents' involvement.

Adult children who become dependent on their parents for one kind of support or another also worry about the impact of their disability on their parents' lives. Knowing that their parents had their own plans and dreams for retirement, they often feel guilty over the disruption they may be causing. Adult children may also worry about their inability to provide the household, financial, or care giving assistance that elderly parents sometimes need. Who will be able to help their parents when and if the need arises? Will other siblings be asked to take on more than their share of the responsibilities? How will they feel about that? Will the parents need to look beyond the family for the help they require?

Disabled adults who return to their parents' home also experience anxiety about the future. Needing to rely on elderly parents for support or care giving makes people feel very vulnerable. Who will be there to help me in the future? How will I have enough money to get the care I need? Will I be alone? Will I have to go into a nursing home? These feelings of anxiety and vulnerability can sometimes cause equally strong feelings of anger and resentment against the very people upon whom one is dependent. No one likes to feel vulnerable. The gradual buildup of these complicated emotions can stress even the most comfortable and loving parent-child relationships.

Reactions of Parents

No MATTER HOW old a child is when he or she becomes disabled, mothers and fathers experience a complex array of feelings ranging from love, concern, and anxiety, to guilt, bitterness, and resentment. Even in parents whose children are fully-grown and independent, the onset of illness and disability can easily rekindle earlier feelings of maternal or paternal protectiveness. They want to keep their child safe from harm and do whatever they can to ensure that he or she will be all right. Watching their child cope with a progressive disease can be a very painful experience for parents, their inability to protect and defend the child causing them to feel helpless, frustrated, and often guilt-ridden. Knowing that genetic susceptibility is a factor in MS, some parents also worry that they somehow caused their child to become disabled and wonder what they could have done to prevent it.

Parents may find themselves, in their middle or later years, providing some combination of living quarters, financial support, physical care, or emotional support to an adult child whom they had once assumed would be independent and part of a family of his or her own. They may feel fortunate to be able to offer one or more of these types of support, while at the same time resenting the disruption of their well-deserved retirement, and worrying about the impact on their own health and financial security.

Parents may also feel resentment toward a child's spouse who has left the marital relationship and "returned" the disabled spouse to the home and care of the parents; although a spouse's role can be ended, the parent feels like a parent forever. This change is sometimes further complicated by grandchildren who, because of their parent's disabilities, may need more than the usual amount of grandparenting. In this situation the grandparents face the delicate challenge of finding a way to participate in the care and nurturance of their grandchildren without overstepping the boundary between grandparent and parent.

Aging parents may suddenly find themselves concerned about the financial security of a child (and grandchildren) they had always assumed would be independent. The world of insurance, government subsidies, trusts, and taxes can be overwhelming to even the most financially astute. Parents, like everyone else, tend to put off thinking about money and the future simply because it is too stressful to do so. Fortunately, there are resources to help with the kind of financial planning that can protect the security of a disabled child and relieve some of this stress (see Chapter 12).

Who Is Taking Care of Whom?

WHETHER THE DISABLED adult is living on his or her own or has returned to the parents' home, certain issues begin to emerge. Parents who are concerned about their child's welfare want what is best for that child. Unfortunately, parents and children do not always agree, no matter how old the child is. Parents may be convinced, for example, that their child should consult a particular physician, take a certain kind of medication, receive a certain type of physical therapy, or get counseling. They may become increasingly anxious, frustrated, and angry when their child does not listen to their advice, even though that child is an adult who is perfectly capable of consulting with doctors, reading the available literature, and making educated choices. These parents feel that they are being asked to stand by and watch their child's condition worsen when, if the child would "just listen," he or she would be better off. This is most often wishful thinking on the part of the parents, but it demonstrates the power of parents' needs to protect and defend their children.

The disabled adult who returns to the parental home may feel as closely supervised as when he or she was a child. Parents' fears often cover a broad spectrum, from physical safety to nutritional health, and from financial responsibility to moral issues. Even an adult child who has been managing these areas of his or her life for a number of years will often find that parents have (strong) opinions, and may express them, about even the most personal issues. This results in part from the parents' natural anxiety about their child, and in part because parents feel—and reasonably so—that anyone living in their home needs to follow the rhythms and "rules" of the household. These feelings can become intermingled in a complex way when significant impairment—either physical or cognitive—is an issue. Parents may worry anew about such things as the child's ability to drive safely, deal with excessive fatigue, handle the effects of alcohol, make responsible decisions, or manage personal finances. Similar to the teenage years, many parents cannot rest peacefully at night until they know that their child is safe at home. The adult child who is accustomed to being able to determine his or her own schedule may suddenly be expected to be home (alone) by a certain hour.

Parent-child boundaries can become particularly blurred in the face of MS-related cognitive impairment. Because the person with MS may, over the course of the disease, experience changes in various cognitive abilities, including memory, attention and concentration, problem-solving, judgment, and spatial orientation (see Chapter 2), parents may become concerned and wonder to what degree they should become involved in, or try to oversee, their child's daily life. Although legal guardianship of the adult child becomes necessary in only the most severe instances of cognitive impairment, some degree of parental guidance may be advisable even with less severe deficits. A thorough evaluation of the cognitive impairment by a neuropsychologist can provide the person with MS and his or her parents with the information they need to determine how involved the parents might need to be. Family counseling can also be helpful to families who are trying to negotiate the delicate balance involved in this situation.

Sometimes, as a result of the anxiety and guilt they feel about their child's MS, parents may have difficulty setting limits on their efforts to care for, help, and protect. Putting all of their own needs, interests, and activities on hold, the parents pursue care-giving activities at the expense of their own health and general well being. Parents need to maintain a balance between the needs of their child with MS and their own needs as individuals and as a couple. This, again, is an area in which family counseling can help to ensure that everyone's needs receive some attention.

Renegotiating the Parent–Child Relationship

PARENTS AND THEIR adult child with MS need to redefine their ongoing relationship in such a way that the feelings and needs of each person can be recognized, accepted, and, to the degree possible, accommodated. For this to occur, these mixed-generation adults must be able to talk about the current situation and the ways in which their roles as parent and child can be adapted or molded to fit the present needs. This is a challenging task for even the most close-knit families.

Empathy, creativity, flexibility, tolerance, and a sense of humor are important ingredients in this type of renegotiation. Parents need to be able to accept and respect the autonomy of their adult child while at the same time offering whatever kinds of support they feel comfortable giving. Adults who have MS need to learn how to express their own needs while simultaneously recognizing their parents' needs and feelings.

"I know you're worried about me but it's uncomfortable to have you asking me how I am all the time; I'm fine right now and I just want to forget about the MS for a while" might be the response of a 25-year-old son who was recently diagnosed and feels smothered by an anxious parent's repeated questions about his health. His parents, in turn, might explain to him that it will take them some time to get accustomed to this frightening and unexpected change in his life, and ask that he keep them up-to-date on how he is doing.

"I know you only want what is best for me, but I need to listen to my doctor's recommendations and make this decision myself"

might be the response of a 38-year-old daughter with MS to parents who are urging her to try a medication they read about in the newspaper or make a visit to a faith healer. Parents who are anxious to help their child get better may want that child to try anything and everything that they hear about from friends or read about in the media. When their well-meaning advice is not followed, the parents may feel hurt, frustrated, rejected, and angry. They need some reassurance that their child has chosen a doctor with expertise in the treatment of MS who will make sure that everything possible is being done to manage symptoms and control disease progression.

"I feel as though you're checking up on me all the time; if I need help I promise I'll call you, but for now I'm doing very well and want to get on with my life" might be the response to parents who call their son many times a week at home or at work to make sure that everything is OK. While the son needs to understand his parents' anxiety and concerns for his welfare, the parents need to understand that he does not want to be treated like a sick person who is unable to take care of himself. He is trying to learn how to live with MS without allowing it to take more time and attention than it really needs.

"Steve has really been very supportive, helping me out more around the house and with the kids' activities. I know you don't think anyone could take as good care of me as you would, but he's doing a great job and I want you to stop criticizing him. It's hurting his feelings and it's no good for our relationship" might be the way a daughter would explain to her parents that she and her husband are adapting well to the demands of MS and that the parents' suggestions might not be as helpful as they intend them to be. She understands that her parents are worried about her, but wants them to realize that she and her husband need to work out their own way of coping with MS.

"I know you're an adult who's used to being on her own, but you need to understand that because of your balance problems I worry when you're out late and I don't know where you are. Please call

and let me know when you plan to be home so I won't need to stay up worrying" might be a parent's request to a daughter who wants to be free to come and go as she pleases in her parents' house. An adult child who returns to the parents' home needs to realize that the parental role is never an easy one to shed. In order to be able to relax and go on with their own lives, the parents may need to know the child's anticipated plans and schedule. In return, of course, the parents should show their child the same courtesy so that he or she does not have to worry about them.

"Please don't be offended if I don't go out to dinner with you and Dad. Since I've moved back in with you, time alone in the house is sometimes the thing I miss most in my life. I'll go out with you next week" might let a parent know that the person misses the privacy he used to take for granted when he lived in his own apartment. Once the privacy issue is openly discussed, it becomes easier for both generations in the household to get on with their lives without feeling offended or worrying about offending the other. Enjoying time together and enjoying time apart can both be part of family life.

"Mom and I are happy to have you here with us, but we need to ask you to pick up after yourself and pitch in a bit—we get tired too" might be said by a father who feels that his grown daughter has settled back a bit too comfortably into a dependent child role. Just as parents may tend to slip easily into an overly protective role with an adult child, a 25- or 35-year-old may find it tempting to be cared for, coddled, and picked up after. Families need to come to some agreement about the shared responsibilities in the household, keeping in mind the schedules, ages, and physical abilities and limitations of each family member.

"Mom, I know that you are concerned about me and my family, and want to help as much as you can, but sometimes it feels as though you're taking over everything. It's important for me to continue doing as many things for my family and myself as I'm still

able to do—even if I have to do it more slowly than you could do it. I promise I'll let you know when I need help" might be said by a daughter whose mother has begun doing so much around her daughter's home that the young woman feels as though she's losing her role as mother and wife. Older parents—particularly those who are retired, may step into the care-giving role so completely that they unwittingly deprive their adult child of the satisfaction of doing things independently.

In each of these examples, parents and children are trying to achieve some balance in meeting their respective needs. There is some recognition on the part of the person making the request of what the other person might be feeling. This kind of thoughtful, empathic, and honest communication will ease the way as family members try to redefine their day-to-day relationship.

Recommendations

▶ *Talk to one another.* It is important to get the feelings and concerns out on the table where you can figure out what to do about them. Family members are sometimes so concerned about hurting one another's feelings that they say nothing at all. Feelings that go unspoken tend to build up, with the result that unidentified tensions pervade the family's relationships and tempers begin to flare. Families who find it too difficult to start this kind of discussion may find that family counseling is an effective way to get the process started.

▶ *Negotiate solutions.* Try to find solutions that are reasonable for all concerned. For this kind of negotiation to happen successfully, family members need to take the time to express their own needs and listen attentively to the needs of others.

▶ *Learn from others.* Chapter events and support groups sponsored by the National MS Society, books and articles, and the Internet are all mechanisms for connecting with other families who are living with MS. They provide opportunities for families to learn from each other's problem-solving efforts while simultaneously offering invaluable emotional support.

▶ *Deal with financial issues frankly and openly.* There is ample help available, from both professionals in the community and written materials, for families' financial planning efforts. Financial worries can be a major source of family tension and upheaval. It is important to find ways to enhance each person's financial security, and it is never too early to start this planning process.

▶ *Share the responsibilities.* Adults sharing a home need to share responsibility for the care and management of that household. Except in the case of very extreme disability, every person can make some useful contribution. Divide responsibilities according to taste, time, and physical ability so that each adult can feel like an important member of the household. There will inevitably be differences of opinion about how various things should be done; these too can be negotiated with some mixture of tolerance, flexibility, and a sense of humor.

▶ *Share the care giving.* Everyone can use some care giving, whether disabled or not. Each member of the family, whether elderly (and possibly disabled) or younger and disabled, needs the care and attention of others. Look for ways to give to one another so that each person can feel that he or she is on both the giving and receiving ends of a caring and supportive relationship.

▶ *Protect everyone's privacy.* Parents and children who are living together need to ensure that everyone has some time, space, activities, and relationships that are separate and theirs alone. Parents need time to themselves and with their friends, and so do adult children. Too much togetherness eventually leads to conflict and resentment. Even the most disabled person who requires a great deal of hands-on care and attention needs some private space and time.

▶ *There is no need to wait for a crisis before seeking help.* Renegotiating the parent-child relationship is never an easy job. It usually requires a significant amount of adjustment on the part of everyone involved. Family members often feel that they should be able to manage these changes without any difficulty simply because they love one another. But it is precisely because family members love one another that the necessary communication and negotiation can become so difficult. When the diagnosis or progression of MS begins to alter the ongoing parent-child relationship, it may be helpful to sit down with a family therapist and talk about the feelings and questions that each family member has and the types of problems they anticipate. This type of discussion and joint problem solving can often resolve tensions before they turn into crises.

▶ *Make full use of available resources.* Living with MS can be exhausting for everyone—including the person who has the disease and those who are helping with care and support. To ensure optimal health and well being for everyone in the family, take advantage of the various types of assistance options your community has to offer; no family needs to do this alone. Chapter 10 offers information about long-term care options and planning. Your chapter of the National MS Society (Call 1-800-FIGHT-MS; 800-344-4867) can guide you in the direction of important community resources.

ADDITIONAL READINGS

Coyle PK, Halper J. *Meeting the Challenges of Progressive Multiple Sclerosis.* New York: Demos Medical Publishing, 2001.

Kalb R, Miller D. In: Kalb R, (ed.) *Multiple Sclerosis: The Questions You Have; The Answers You Need* (3rd ed.). New York: Demos Medical Publishing, 2004.

Russell LM, Grant AE. *The Life Planning Workbook: A Hands-On Guide to Help Parents Provide for the Future Security and Happiness of Their Child with Disability After Their Death.* Evanston, IL: American Publishing Company, 1995.

Russell LM, Grant AE, Joseph SM, Fee RW. *Planning for the Future: Providing a Meaningful Life for a Child with a Disability After Your Death* (2nd ed.) Evanston, IL: American Publishing, 1995.

9

The Caregiving Relationship

Deborah Miller, Ph.D.
Peggy Crawford, Ph.D.

THIS CHAPTER EXPLORES the challenges faced by individuals with *moderate* to *severe* multiple sclerosis (MS) and their care giving partners, when the disease progresses to the point that the person with MS needs significant amounts of help with daily routines and personal care activities. The types of help and care most often needed by people who have significant disability are described, the changes that can result in the relationship when the partner or partner provides that care are discussed, and ways to manage those changes are recommended. Although relatively few families living with MS will find themselves dealing with this level of disability, the chapter is intended to help those families step back a bit—perhaps to view their situation from a somewhat different perspective—and to consider options for helping themselves and their loved ones.

In the most ideal of circumstances, families living with severe MS approach their inter-relationships as a *care partnership*, in which each person is involved in many aspects of family life, including managing MS-related changes. The term *care partners* encourages individuals to think of themselves as working together to create and implement management solutions and problem-solving strategies. In addition, it suggests the importance of considering the needs and wants of everyone involved—not just those of the person with MS.

When MS results in significant physical and/or cognitive disability, or one care partner's emotional reaction or adjustment to the disease is totally out of sync with that of other family members, the partnership may become imbalanced or out of kilter. The ways in which a partnership can become imbalanced and the feelings this can cause, as well as strategies for protecting the balance and restoring it when it has been lost are described. Also, some suggestions for making the situation livable in the event that the imbalance cannot be corrected are presented. Because this chapter focuses primarily on couples that are living with MS, the person with the disease is referred to as the MS-partner, and the person who does not have MS is called the well partner. Another term, caregiver, is used specifically for those who provide help with personal care or daily routines.

Care Partner Characteristics

APPROXIMATELY ONE-QUARTER OF the 400,000 people with MS in the United States require help with daily activities or personal care. They receive most of their help from partners, who typically have major additional responsibilities, including employment and childcare. People who have disabling MS tend to be married and in their forties and fifties by the time they need help with daily routines. Their significant disability is the result of physical symptoms, cognitive changes, or some combination of both. Approximately one-third of people with MS have difficulty walking without assistance. Some face increasing dependence for personal care, toileting, home management, and getting around in their homes and communities. Regardless of their physical condition, approximately 10% of people with MS have cognitive problems that are significant enough to interfere with various activities of daily living.

The families living with this stage of MS typically have children in their teens, who are preparing to leave home or already out on their own. There may also be aging parents, themselves in need of increasing amounts of assistance from their adult children.

"Old Hands" at Multiple Sclerosis

THE FAMILIES DESCRIBED in this chapter have generally been living with MS for a significant amount of time. They have already managed many MS-related changes, in a gradual process that began when they learned that a family member had a chronic illness that could cause increasing disability. These families have had more contact with healthcare providers and insurance companies than most people. They have had to learn about the many symptoms that MS can produce and how those symptoms can change over time. Family members have also gotten over the hurdle of "going public," because the MS-partner typically has visible symptoms that require the use of an ambulation aid. Extended family and friends have become involved, perhaps by helping the MS-partner in some way or by providing emotional support for a member of the family.

Living with unpredictability has become a way of life, and everyone in the family has had numerous experiences with having to change or cancel long-awaited plans because of the disease. The MS-partner has probably had to limit or stop working outside the home or performing many household chores. The family has dealt with loss of income and the ongoing presence of the MS-partner around the house. They have learned to pitch in with the housekeeping or maintenance chores that the MS-partner previously handled. There have been other noticeable changes in the routines of family life as well. The couple has probably changed how they spend their free time, both individually and together. They have undoubtedly thought about how they will handle the future, when and if things begin to change dramatically.

Types of Help People Need

EVEN WITH THE many adaptations they have already made, well-partners may find it difficult to keep up with the caregiving responsibilities that face them on a daily basis. Keep in mind that it is generally not the major, short-term crises or stresses that people find most challenging; it seems, instead, to be the ongoing, low-grade pressures of daily life that produce the biggest stress.

Some of the common problems related to progressive MS—unsafe mobility, bladder and bowel incontinence, and the behavioral changes that can come with cognitive problems—are known to be particularly stressful for caregivers. In order to manage these problems and the stress that they can cause, it is useful to think about the different kinds of help that well-partners provide. This enables the well-partner to evaluate the caregiving situation and (1) think about how best to manage the physical activities involved in caregiving, (2) figure out why certain aspects of the situation seem especially stressful, and (3) sort out the kinds of help that may be available from family, friends, or paid help.

Hands-On (Instrumental) Help

THE MOST OBVIOUS type of assistance provided by well-partners is called *instrumental* or *hands-on* help. This includes activities that take place each day at predictable times (e.g., helping the MS-partner bathe and dress in the morning, take medications, or get ready for bed). Other hands-on activities, like helping the MS-partner move from one chair to another or get to the bathroom, refilling an empty drink cup, or getting something from another room, happen often but at unpredictable times during the day and night. Still other hands-on help occurs at planned but less frequent intervals (e.g., assisting with nail care or correspondence, traveling to medical appointments, and shopping).

Planning And Decision-Making

OVER THE COURSE of their relationship, couples generally come to a working agreement regarding those issues that they decide together and those that they handle individually. Helping a partner gather information and make important decisions happens at one time or another in virtually all relationships. Regardless of their previous way of doing things, however, well-partners generally must become very involved in gathering information and making decisions with or for a significantly disabled MS-partner. This may be because of the physical symptoms of the person with

MS, such as visual impairment, or cognitive symptoms, such as difficulties with remembering or arriving at a reasonable decision.

It becomes increasingly important for well-partners to be involved in treatment planning as they become responsible for implementing various parts of the plan. It may be the well-partner who manages the medication schedule, gives a drug injection, or performs intermittent bladder catheterization. Treatment plans can fail if the well-partner does not know the medical staff or have their ready support, does not understand why and how a procedure is done, or is simply told to carry out treatment routines that are completely incompatible with his or her schedule.

Emotional Support

IN ADDITION TO help with daily activities and decision making, people with significant disability need ongoing emotional support. As in most lasting, intimate relationships, they look to partners for understanding, respect, reassurance, and encouragement.

How Caregiving Impacts the Couple's Relationship

AT THE HEART of most long-term relationships are mutual concern, respect, and affection; an enjoyment of each other's company; and a shared history as well as hopes and plans for the future. Although these aspects of commitment are just as important for couples that are living with advanced disability, there are inevitable shifts in some aspects of the relationship. The need to give and receive intimate personal care, the well-partner's irritation at always being on call, and the MS-partner's frustration at having to wait for help or concern over being a bother inevitably have an impact on the couple's emotional life. For some well-partners (particularly those whose MS-partners have experienced significant cognitive changes), the emotional investment gradually shifts from being a romantic commitment, a shared raising of their children, and planning for a healthy future, to one that is based on friendship, managing the current situation ("getting through the day"), and a commitment to keeping the marriage vows. Even in the face of this shift in feelings, the emotional support provided by the well-partner becomes increasingly essential to the MS-partner, whose social network tends to grow narrower.

The MS-partner's increasing dependence and need for various kinds of help bring about inevitable changes in the marital relationship. These changes may happen slowly over an extended period of time or abruptly because of sudden disease activity. Some couples report that the disease has gradually allowed them to make room for the disability and related caregiving activities in their relationship and family life. "Taking things as they come" has become the family motto, and the adaptation has been relatively comfortable. Not surprisingly, however, many couples find that unexpected changes remain unwanted challenges. The changes often come during the family's peak years of career and family responsibilities and seem to affect all aspects of family life.

Some people believe that there is no point in thinking about or discussing these stresses because there is little that can be done about them. They acknowledge that they got the short straw in the "in sickness and in health" gamble. Our experience as clinicians and caregivers, however, is quite the opposite. By increasing their awareness of the specific situations that cause stress and examining how they have successfully managed changes in the past, couples can devise strategies for enhancing the care partnership while minimizing caregiver burn-out.

Caregiver Strain and Stress

CAREGIVER BURN-OUT HAS many different causes, including *physical strain* and *emotional stress*. The physical strain results from the variety of hands-on activities that are required of the caregiver and the fact that these activities are superimposed on other commitments and responsibilities. Emotional stress comes from the well-partner's reactions to providing care and to unwanted changes in his or her own lifestyle, as well as from the reactions of the MS-partner to receiving care. These stresses and strains can, in turn, cause physical and emotional health problems for the partner caregiver.

The physical strains experienced by the well-partner are most directly linked to the physical and cognitive problems of the MS-partner. The greater the disability, the more hands-on care is required. This can involve such activities as lifting the MS-partner several times a day, cleaning up after bladder or bowel accidents, and getting wheelchairs in and out of cars.

In contrast, the emotional stress of caregivers seems to have little to do with the physical condition of the MS-partner or the length of time the partner has been disabled. Emotional stress seems more related to how "trapped" well-partners feel in their situation. This, in turn, seems to be closely related to the level of satisfaction they have in their marriages. Additional factors may include the degree to which well-partners and MS-partners agree about MS and related care needs, how well the MS-partner is coping emotionally with the illness, the extent of cognitive impairment, and the amount of time available to the well-partner to pursue personal interests and activities. Most often, the greatest distress for the well-partner is caused by the emotional stress that comes with the decision-making and emotional support aspects of caregiving, rather than the physical strain of hands-on care. This is important because most of the problems that cause stress become more manageable when they are better understood.

Before looking at specific areas of stress in greater detail, it may be helpful to address the common concern about divorce in MS (and other chronic illnesses). Many people assume that the pressures and challenges of living with MS inevitably lead to a higher than normal divorce rate. Although there are no exact data on the number of MS marriages that end in divorce, the best available evidence indicates that the rate is actually lower than the 50% divorce rate of the general population in the United States. Apparently, some couples that might otherwise have separated remain together after MS has been diagnosed. Well-partners may stay in a marriage because of a sense of commitment and obligation; MS-partners may remain in an unhappy marriage because of concerns about financial security or insurance benefits.

The important thing to remember is that every long-term intimate relationship has its strengths and weaknesses. In most instances, those strengths and weaknesses existed well before the stresses of MS were added to the picture. The intrusion of MS tends to highlight both the positive and the negative aspects of any relationship. Their relative balance ultimately helps to determine the success with which a couple confronts this new and extraordinary challenge. It is rare for MS to cause a solid and satisfying marriage to fail; it is even less likely to turn a foundering relationship into a successful one.

Some well-partners who feel obliged to honor the marriage commitment may gradually distance themselves from the relationship emotionally, physically, and even financially. In many ways, this pseudo-divorce may be more painful and detrimental to the MS-partner than a legal divorce. For instance, as long as the couple remains together, it may be more difficult or awkward for family and friends to offer or provide help to the MS-partner. In some states, the MS-partner might remain ineligible for certain kinds of community support that would be available to a single person. In the event of a legal divorce, the partners can acknowledge their separation, grieve over the loss of their past relationship, and begin the process of rebuilding their lives. Family members and friends can more easily meet the emotional, financial, and physical needs of the MS-partner. Eligibility for community programs and other benefits can be explored.

Couples who are unable or unwilling to repair a foundering relationship should make every effort to be honest about what is happening and responsible about ensuring that the needs of the MS-partner will be met. As with other difficult life circumstances, the first step in dealing with the problem is admitting its existence; the next step is to find ways to manage it as comfortably as possible for all concerned.

Areas of Stress and Conflict

Seeing MS Through Two Pairs Of Eyes

DIFFERENCES OF OPINION about the amount of care and assistance needed by the MS-partner are a common source of conflict among couples. For example, the MS-partner may feel the need for more help or attention than the well-partner thinks is required.

In this situation, the well-partner may become resentful of the demands being made, whereas the MS-partner interprets the partner's reluctance or resentment as an indication of insensitivity, selfishness, or even emotional abandonment.

Conversely, the caregiver who is concerned about the MS-partner's physical safety, driving skills, or cognitive abilities may feel the need to become more involved in the MS-partner's daily activities than the MS-partner believes is necessary. Some combination of resistance on the part of the MS-partner to acknowledging change or loss of personal abilities, and anxiety on the part of the well-partner can make it difficult to reach any kind of agreement. This situation is particularly stressful because it highlights a shift in the couple's prior relationship—a change from the more "equal" partnership in which each person made personal decisions for himself or herself to a relationship in which the well-partner begins to feel obliged to take on a more managerial or supervisory role.

The Uses Of Time

GRADUALLY, COUPLES LIVING with disabling MS make significant changes in how they use their time, both individually and together. Most of the well-partner's unscheduled time is devoted to the routines of maintaining the household, attending to the children, and managing the MS-partner's care needs. The well-partner often works outside the home and has limited free time. Every minute of the day is full. Errands are done as the opportunity presents and as quickly as possible. The list of things to do in a day is long, and getting through the list is a higher priority than doing the chores well. Children need help with homework and transportation for after-school activities. Any "alone time" is at a premium and needs to be carefully protected.

The MS-partner, on the other hand, may have been home alone all day, looking forward to the partner's company in the evening. Any free time that the well-partner spends reading, exercising, or doing other things that do not include the MS-partner is a disappointment to the partner who has MS. In addition, the MS-partner who becomes increasingly frustrated by his or her inability to perform household chores wants to see them taken care of quickly and thoroughly. When the couple sees each other at the end of the day, there can be a clash of needs for "alone" versus "together" time, or the wish for "a little quiet time" versus the desire to "get some things done." Well-partners frequently describe feeling forced to choose among doing for themselves, meeting their household and family responsibilities, and meeting the needs and hopes of their partners.

The Use Of Space

COUPLES OFTEN HAVE differences of opinion about how much the home should be rearranged or modified to accommodate MS, or whether they should consider moving in order to make life more manageable. Either the caregiver or the MS-partner may be reluctant to have a commode chair in the living room, build a ramp on the front of the house, or give up the family home and move to an accessible condo. These disagreements are usually motivated by a complex set of feelings and needs. They may involve differences of opinion about the best ways to manage the disability, as well as a desire to keep things appearing as normal as possible (especially if there are children at home). In addition, one or another partner may simply "draw the line," because of a feeling that far too much has already been sacrificed to the disease and to the other person's needs. This sense of having reached a limit of personal sacrifice is a common but somewhat embarrassing feeling for people, with the result that it is seldom acknowledged, much less discussed.

The Use Of Financial Resources

MS CAN BE a costly disease. Financial concerns are among some of the most common sources of conflict for any couple. MS-associated costs, including medical care, the available disease-modifying drugs, adaptive equipment, and professional caregiving help, can directly conflict with educational expenses for the children, a car that provides reliable transportation, and saving for retirement. These issues can be a major source of disagreement in a marriage, and they require patience, commitment, and good communication skills for successful resolution (see Chapters 9 and 10).

The Sexual Relationship

INTIMACY AND SEXUALITY can be profoundly affected by chronic illness. Chapter 4 discusses in detail the various ways in which MS can interfere with intimacy and sexual expression. Of particular relevance here, however, is the potential impact of caregiving activities on the well-partner's sexual feelings for his or her MS-partner. Much of the help that well-partners provide involves intimate (but nonsexual) and sometimes unappealing contact. This might include assistance with dressing, bathing, or eating, and catheterizing or cleaning up after an episode of incontinence. Well-partners often describe themselves as "turning off their feelings" when they give that kind of intimate assistance. Then, when they try to be sexual with their partners, well-partners sometimes find that they remain emotionally turned off and disinterested in physical intimacy. The caregiver's near-constant state of fatigue, worry over the growing list of responsibilities, and sadness over changes in the marital relationship have as much impact on the couple's sexual relationship as the changes in sexual function experienced by the MS-partner. These feelings and concerns need to be shared and discussed in order for the relationship to grow in a meaningful and comfortable way.

Feeling Cheated

MS CAN CREATE a deep sense of unfairness in a relationship, leaving one or both of the partners feeling cheated and angry. They may even find themselves locked in a contest over who has it worse. MS-partners tend to believe that their situation is the most uncomfortable, frustrating, and unfair, whereas well-partners feel equally trapped and disabled by an illness that is not even their own. These valid and intense feelings can be difficult to curb, and finding a positive way to deal with them is a significant challenge for many couples. This is especially true if the couple has few friends, family members, or professional helpers to whom they can or are willing to turn. Sometimes in the absence of other outlets, the built-up frustration and anger are directed at each other.

Many MS-partners have described the anger that they have about the disease and the ways that the anger becomes focused on the well-partner who can leave the house at will, decide what food is bought at the grocery store, and even determine when the MS-partner gets up and goes to bed. These MS-partners resent their dependence on their partners. Thus, the anger that a person with MS feels over the limitations imposed by the disease tends to spill over onto the partner who is providing much of the necessary help and care. The well-partner, in turn, feels unfairly targeted by the accumulated anger and resentment.

MS-partners who are severely limited in what they can do on their own sometimes feel a need to reassure themselves that their well-partners are truly there for them. They may test this with frequent requests for help or by calling out to their well-partners "just to check" where they are. Sometimes, the cognitive problems of MS can make it uncontrollably difficult for MS-partners to sort out what has to happen *now* and what can wait. This loss of impulse control can result in well-partners feeling trapped by a situation in which they are "on call 24/7."

Maggie Strong (whose husband had MS) and Jane Bendetson (whose husband was disabled by cardiac disease) of the Well-Partner Foundation write about how disabling it feels to become the working arms and legs for one's partner. These two writers and others have described the way that friends and family members seem to expect that they, as well-partners, will naturally, willingly, and successfully take up the caregiving role when, in fact, this is not always the case. These writers speculate that this expectation results from the fact that family and friends would not know what to do if they were asked to pitch in and help with the care.

When Frustration Leads to Abuse

ALL OF THESE stresses and frustrations, whether they relate to life plans that have been thwarted, unwanted responsibility, or increasing dependency, often have no constructive outlet. It is not uncommon for emotionally harmful behaviors to develop between partners. Hurtful words are spoken during a difficult transfer into the car, shouting matches erupt when the well-partner is late arriving home, doors are slammed when there is a disagreement, or threats are made about putting a hospital bed in the family room, nursing home placement, or divorce. These angry encounters, probably never part of the relationship before MS, may become increasingly common.

Couples who have never raised a hand toward one another in anger may occasionally become physically abusive. Such physically hurtful exchanges usually begin to occur in the context of giving or getting personal help. It can begin in small ways—the well-partner being rough when brushing the MS-partner's hair or giving a bath, or the MS-partner scratching the well-partner during a transfer. Once frustration and anger have reached this point, physical abuse by either partner may become more frequent. There is usually a great deal of very honest guilt and shame after these events, with promises to partner and self that it will never occur again. Often, though, it does recur, perhaps worse than the time before. For that reason alone, no level of abusive behavior is acceptable. While the circumstances that create the frustrations leading to abuse are often unavoidable, the response of physical aggressiveness is not. That is why it is so important to be aware of the tensions as they mount and do something about them before more emotional or physical harm is done.

The majority of couples never experiences such levels of distress or become abusive. It is important to be aware, however, that mutual love, deep commitment, religious values, or financial resources do not necessarily protect partners from becoming hurtful to one another. Outbursts begin to occur when people ignore mounting frustration, fail to recognize that they cannot control themselves, and are unable to identify any options for themselves. The only acceptable position to take is that abusive behavior is never acceptable, and that creating solutions is possible if the couple is willing to admit their stress and seek help. The best way to avoid bringing abuse into the relationship is to prevent the painful emotions that lead to it.

How to Keep the Relationship Alive and Well

Effective Communication

THERE ARE SOME general things that all couples who are dealing with advanced MS can do to keep the care partnership alive and well, and some very specific things. The most important skill for any couple is good communication. Being able to share feelings, opinions, and points of view, by taking the time to talk to and listen to one another, is essential to any successful partnership. Although couples who are not living with chronic illness often rely on communicating "on the run" while sharing a ride to work, gardening, or before they fall asleep, couples who live with MS find that they cannot count on such opportunities. Because of time constraints, fatigue, or MS-related memory, attention, or concentration problems, MS couples may have to work harder than most couples to find the best routine for "staying connected," and making it a routine is very important.

Decisions that need to be made and disagreements that need to be resolved are best dealt with one at a time before they become problems. Couples who have trouble making time to talk together, or find that very intense feelings about several issues have gotten mixed together, should consider consulting a marriage counselor who is familiar with chronic disease. Such a therapist can help the couple work through existing problems and build skills for managing future concerns. This, in turn, can relieve some of the emotional pressure and help make the communication process more productive and enjoyable. Many couples find that knowing a therapist with whom each partner is comfortable, and whom they can consult periodically, is as important as having a good neurologist.

Relieving the Pressures Of Caregiving

EARLIER WE DESCRIBED caregiving as falling into three general kinds of help (instrumental or hands-on, decision making, and emotional support) and suggested that thinking about care in this way could be useful for finding solutions to difficulties. The initial step in creating a solution is to understand the problem and break it down into manageable parts. Then, even if the whole problem cannot be completely resolved, at least some parts can be more comfortably managed. As described, hands-on or instrumental help tends to cause physical strain on the caregiver, whereas the necessary decision making and emotional support tend to be more emotionally stressful.

⊙ Managing instrumental care

A FIRST STEP in figuring out ways to reduce the physical strain of hands-on care is to find out if there is a healthier or easier way to do the job. With a doctor's prescription, most insurance companies will pay for an occupational or physical therapist to make a home visit. This specialist can advise on ways to manage transfers that will protect both the well-partner and the MS-partner; suggest equipment that will make the kitchen, bathroom, and bedroom safer and more accessible; and devise strategies for managing other logistical problems in the household. Couples should not hesitate to discuss home management difficulties with their physician. Symptoms that interfere with daily activities (e.g., spasticity and fatigue), can often be managed with medications or other treatment strategies.

For a variety of reasons, many couples are reluctant to ask family and friends for help. They often feel that help should be offered without their having to ask for it. Sometimes family and friends are interested and willing to help, but do not know how to do so. Or they may be concerned about making commitments that they cannot keep. Couples should take the initiative in asking for help. The worst they can get is a no.

The best strategy is usually to ask family and friends for help with those needs that come at predictable but infrequent times, such as a trip to the doctor or shopping. The request should be a specific one. "Would you be willing to stay with your sister one Saturday so I can run a bunch of errands" is not as likely to get the job done as "I have an appointment with the dentist in two weeks at 1:00, which should take about two hours, including travel time. Would you stay with your sister that day while I'm gone?" This kind of request gives the family member a specific event to help with, an idea of how long it will take, and time to make the necessary arrangements.

It is also possible to recruit people to help with routine but occasional activities that are social in nature as well as instrumental. This might involve asking a neighbor or church member to come in to wash and set the MS-partner's hair on a regular basis. Once family and friends become more comfortable spending time with the MS-partner, they tend to make themselves more available.

Transportation for the MS-partner is often a major worry. Many chapters of the National MS Society and other community agencies help people travel to and from medical appointments. Some community transit authorities have programs for their disabled customers. These options should be explored, perhaps by a family member who has mentioned, "if there is ever anything I can do. . . ."

The caregiving that is done daily at planned times can be difficult and demanding for well-partners. It is unlikely, however, that family and friends can routinely provide this kind of help because of their own schedules and commitments. Some couples find that it is worthwhile to hire help, either through an agency or privately. Most state departments of human services offer a Home and Community Waiver program that makes home health aides and other services available. Eligibility requirements and programs differ from state to state but should be investigated with a social worker, the National MS Society, or the county department of human services. Family members may differ in their feelings about having strangers in the home to provide personal care, but the fact remains that competent assistance is often available and having that assistance can help preserve the health and well-being of the partner caregiver and possibly the marital relationship.

In many respects, unpredictable daily needs are the most emotionally stressful for couples, and they tend to leave the well-partner feeling either trapped or constantly "on call," to *help* or *get* or *find* or *do* one thing or another. Since these unpredictable requests can result from emotional needs as well as physical limitations, the responses of the well-partner can become quite emotional as well. It is important for a couple to talk together about how they are each reacting to the other's needs and to discuss the best ways to manage those reactions. Providing the MS-partner with the security of a portable telephone or emergency alert service may ease the tension both partners feel when the well-partner is away from home. Day respite programs are offered by some MS comprehensive care centers and other community agencies. Such programs can be a valuable alternative to staying home alone, especially for those who require frequent help and a structured environment. There is no single solution to matters of managing the "hands on" care needs. Developing a workable solution comes from working together to understand what needs to be done, being open-minded about the possibilities for getting the job done, and balancing each partner's needs.

⊙ Managing decision-making and emotional support needs

THE EFFORTS OF well-partners to meet the decision-making and emotional support needs of their partners, as well as their own reactions to caregiving, require as much creativity and energy as hands-on care. The greatest source of that energy is a satisfying marital relationship. Well-partners who are in satisfying marriages experience less emotional distress, regardless of the kinds of help they are required to provide. It follows from this that some of the best caregiving medicine is to keep or make the marriage healthy. Most marriages have a trouble spot or two that seem manageable until the additional challenge of MS enters the picture. In order for a couple to get along, it is essential to keep those trouble spots from becoming open wounds. This is best done by acknowledging the difficulties and devising solutions. Some couples choose to handle these issues on their own, whereas others opt to work with a marriage counselor or attend a couples' support group, such as those offered by many National MS Society chapters or comprehensive care clinics.

Couples living with severely disabling MS sustain many significant losses during their lives. These may include having to give up activities they enjoy doing together, changing career goals, being unable to provide for their children as they had planned, or having difficulty planning for retirement. Couples who are successful at managing these losses and remaining committed to one another seem to do so by recognizing the need to be in charge of MS, rather than the other way around, and by seeking help and tapping available resources along the way. In order to turn losses into challenging opportunities, couples need to give their marriage and family first priority, and they must be willing to work MS into the rest of their lives.

Having a plan for the future can be an important part of this process. Many couples begin to live one day at a time, in part to avoid the frightening realities that the future may hold. Having a plan can help put worries to rest and prepare people to be more in control, no matter what the future brings. Occasionally, the physical and cognitive problems of MS can be so advanced that the well-partner must take over all decision making for the MS-partner. Such severe disability can be very distressing for the well-partner who is grieving the loss of his or her formerly equal partner. This situation can be somewhat easier to manage if the couple has been able to talk and plan together well in advance. An open discussion of this kind enables the well-partner to understand the wishes of the MS-partner and take them into account in treatment and long-term care decisions (e.g., nursing home placement or life-sustaining treatments). Life-planning issues are described in detail in Chapter 12.

Conclusion

WELL-PARTNERS WHO ARE caregivers for loved ones with disabling MS have many responsibilities. Among the most critical are keeping themselves and their relationship healthy. This involves attending to their personal health and emotional needs; working with their partners to manage problems in the relationship; recognizing that everyone has a limit to what he or she can bear; and knowing what their own limits are. Well-partners need friends, hobbies, and other social and emotional outlets, and they need to recognize that asking for help is a sign of honesty and strength. It may also mean making sure that they have their own

MS-free zone in the home—a place where they can feel "off duty," if only for short periods of time. Taking these steps will help partners maintain their *care partnership*—in the true sense of the word—and ensure the well-being of their partners and themselves. Taking charge in this way can help put MS in its place and keep family life as the central focus.

ADDITIONAL READINGS

National MS Society Publications
　　(available by calling 1-800-FIGHT-MS (1-800-344-4867) or
　　online at http://www.nationalmssociety.org/library.asp)
Harmon, J. At Home with MS: Adapting Your Environment.
Redford T. A Guide for Caregivers.
Hiring Help at Home: The Basic Facts.
Minden L, Frankel D. PLAINTALK: A Booklet About MS for Families.
Brown SM. So You Have Progressive MS.

GENERAL READINGS

Carroll DL, Dudley J, Dorman JD. *Living Well with MS: A Guide for Patient, Caregiver, and Family.* New York: HarperCollins, 1993.

Cohen MD. *Dirty Details.* Philadelphia: Temple University Press, 1996.

Coyle PK, Halper J. *Meeting the Challenges of Progressive Multiple Sclerosis.* New York: Demos Medical Publishing, 2001.

Frankel D. Long-term care. In: Kalb R, (ed.) *Multiple Sclerosis: The Questions You Have; The Answers You Need* (3rd ed.) New York: Demos Medical Publishing, 2004.

Holland N, Halper J, (eds.) Multiple Sclerosis: A Self-Care Guide to Wellness (2nd ed). New York: Demos Medical Publishing, 2004.

Kalb R, Miller D. Psychosocial issues. In: Kalb R, (ed.) *Multiple Sclerosis: The Questions You Have; The Answers You Need* (3rd ed.). New York: Demos Medical Publishing, 2004.

Kaufman M, Silverberg C, Odette F. The Ultimate Guide to Sex and Disability. San Francisco: Cleis Press, 2003.

Mintz SB. Love, Honor, and Value: A Family Caregiver Speaks out about the Choices and Challenges of Caregiving. Capital Books, Inc., 2002.

Price J. Avoiding Attendants from Hell: A Practical Guide to Funding, Hiring, and Keeping Personal Care Attendants. Science and Humanities Press, 1998. [www.banis-associates.com]

Schwarz SP. 300 Tips for Making Life with Multiple Sclerosis Easier. New York: Demos Medical Publishing, 1999.

Strong M. Mainstay: For the Well Spouse of the Chronically Ill. Bradford Books, 1997.

10

Planning Wisely For Possible Care Needs

Dorothy Northrop, MSW

Introduction

LOOKING AHEAD AND planning for the future can be an exciting and exhilarating experience. We anticipate and busily plan for graduations, weddings, new babies, new homes, or job promotions. Planning for happy events makes us feel good. On the other hand, looking to the future and anticipating the possibility of illness or disability, as well as the eventuality of old age, is more likely to be uncomfortable, stressful, and unsettling. Because of the discomfort involved, it is tempting to avoid this unpleasantness and stop what many would describe as pessimistic and morbid thinking.

If anticipating and planning for the unknowns and negative eventualities of life make people so uncomfortable, how do we motivate ourselves to turn our thoughts in this direction? How do we overcome our anxieties and turn the process into something that is reassuring and affirming? This is not an easy task for anyone, but once the planning process is underway, it can bring a sense of mastery and control to one's future, and a confidence in one's ability to meet whatever turns and detours lie ahead.

Fortunately, we live in a time when planning for the future and anticipating the support one might need to remain active and independent are receiving increasing public attention. With modern medicine and the technological advances of recent years, life expectancy in our society is the highest that it has ever been. Where previously families tended to provide the safety net of care for their members, today's fragmented and mobile population means that many families are not available to assume this role. In addition, many households depend on the employment of all adult family members in order to meet expenses, a reality that certainly impacts the availability of family support. When you add to this scenario the rising cost of purchasing assistance and services, it is understandable why our society is beginning to give increasing attention to long-term care insurance, financial planning, elder law specialization, and various other strategies to anticipate and address future care needs.

This chapter is designed to help you think comfortably and constructively about the long-term care needs that a person with MS might encounter. Could there be a time when you or a family member with MS might need help with personal care such as dressing, bathing, transferring, or toileting? What about meal preparation, grocery shopping, laundry, housekeeping, or money management? Although it is advisable for everyone—with or without MS—to anticipate a future decline in health and avoid crises through careful life planning, living with a chronic, variable, and unpredictable disease such as MS makes this endeavor even more critical. In addition, once a diagnosis of MS has been established, options such as the purchase of disability insurance and/or long-term care insurance may no longer be available. Alternative creative and thoughtful strategies will need to be explored (see Chapter 12).

Although finding such alternatives may seem a daunting task, it is seldom the development of the plan that is the most challenging aspect of this process. What can be even more difficult is addressing the anxiety and fear that can come with that planning, and moving from seeing such planning as "giving in" to the disease, to seeing the planning process as the vehicle by which choices will be assured and quality of life maintained.

Planning as a Family

FAMILIES LIVING WITH MS benefit most when all family members engage in the planning process together. If the person with MS experiences functional decline, what resources could be pulled together to ensure that he or she could continue to be actively involved in family activities and community life? What kinds of equipment, home modifications, personal assistance, household help, and transportation services will be needed? How many of these needs can family members meet? When will outside resources be required? Who will arrange for these resources? How much will they cost?

People quickly find, as they embark on this kind of dialogue, that not all family members think alike. Members of a family will approach this kind of discussion from very different perspectives. They are at different places in their lives in terms of age, experience, responsibilities, life plans, needs, strengths, and emotional make-up. They will cope differently when asked to think about a day when their loved one may need more hands-on assistance in order to compensate for physical decline. Some will become anxious and want to avoid the topic. Others might want to jump in and start detailed planning right away. Some will be very flexible in their thinking and not have strong opinions, one way or the other. Others will have very strong ideas about how to go forward.

As with many other family issues, it will take time and perseverance to see the process through, but such a dialogue will undoubtedly result in a plan that will be the most realistic and have the best chance for success. If your family finds it too difficult or stressful to initiate these conversations, you might wish to meet with a family counselor to help you jumpstart the process. Your chapter of the National MS Society can refer you to counselors in your area who are familiar with MS and long-term planning issues.

The important thing to remember is that there is no right or wrong solution to this planning discussion. Every family is different. Every family has access to different resources. Finances vary. Family members have different strengths, abilities, needs, and priorities. Community services and programs vary through-out the country. Since it is only the family members who know best what will work in their particular situation(s), non-participation in this kind of discussion puts them at a great dis-advantage and limits options and choices.

Topics for Family Discussion

CHOICE and CONSUMER DIRECTION are becoming the operative words in addressing long-term care needs. Long-term care is no longer a phrase associated only with nursing home care; it refers to a continuum of care that includes a range of services in a variety of settings—the home, day programs, assisted living facilities, as well as nursing homes. This continuum of care can begin at any age, and be provided by both formal (professional) and informal (non-professional) caregivers. Therefore, being knowledgeable consumers of long-term care services requires that families be aware of their needs and informed about their options. To begin the process, it is important to have adequate information in the following areas:

- ▶ Potential impact of MS
- ▶ Individual needs and priorities within the family
- ▶ Availability of public and private resources
- ▶ Potential uses of adaptive equipment and assistive technology
- ▶ Advantages and disadvantages of various long-term care options
- ▶ Financial resources.

Potential Impact of MS

IN ORDER TO be able to communicate effectively with each other and with potential resources in the community, family members need to be knowledgeable about MS—both in terms of the needs it is generating right now and its potential impact down the road. Keeping a healthcare journal can help the person with MS monitor his or her health and well-being, while tracking any health-

or disability-related needs; a frank and open discussion with one's physician can be helpful in anticipating long-term medical needs.

Individual Needs and Priorities within the Family

WHEN LOOKING TO the future, the thoughts and concerns of the person with MS must be central to the discussion. What are his or her goals? Which interests and activities have priority? What are his or her values? Does the person prioritize independence or safety? Self-sufficiency or being cared for? Privacy or socialization? Being careful or taking risks? Once issues such as these are understood, it will be clearer how to proceed in the planning.

It is also important in any discussion regarding the future that assumptions held by both the person with MS and family members are put openly on the table and discussed. For example, perhaps the family member with MS has always assumed that loved ones would be there to meet his or her needs, whether it be administering medications, running errands, cleaning the house, or providing hands-on assistance. What may work in the present, however, may be problematic down the road when children have moved away and a spouse's health has declined. In the same way, family members might assume there will never be a time when they would not be available to assist their loved one, failing to leave room for unanticipated life events, career demands, significant health issues, and inadequate community support services.

Community Resources

UNTIL THE NEED arises, most families are completely unaware of the many kinds of resources that are available in the community to help meet their needs. Talking about needs that might arise in the future—and looking into possible options for meeting them—allows time to identify potential resources and formal options of support, including state and county programs, VA programs, paratransit services, and providers of home health, adult day programs, assisted living, and skilled nursing care. Being knowledgeable about the support systems that are available puts a family many steps ahead if and when such services are required.

Identifying resources and making choices in a crisis situation is difficult and often less effective; having a well-thought-out contingency plan helps families feel more secure, prepared, and in control.

Adaptive Equipment and Assistive Technology

ASSISTIVE TECHNOLOGY REFERS to all of the tools, products, and devices—from the simplest gadgets to the most complex mobility aids and computer systems—which can make it easier and safer for a person to function and for caregivers to provide assistance. Becoming familiar with assistive technology resources enables families to enhance accessibility and safety within the home and the community, and evaluate the resources available in other long-term care settings.

Long-Term Care Options: Advantages and Disadvantages

WHEN CONSIDERING THE various options available for long-term care, it is important for families to have a clear picture of what each has to offer, as well as what the potential drawbacks might be. This allows family members to discuss which of the alternatives is best suited to their needs including:

▶ *Home Care*: Many services can be brought into the home to support family living. However, issues such as the shortage of home health aides, the cost of such aides, the difficulty of accessing services in rural areas, and home safety must be considered.

▶ *Adult Day Programs*: Day programs are usually located in the community and are relatively low cost. They provide socialization for the participant as well as respite for the caregiver. However, many of the programs are elderly-focused; wheelchairs and incontinence may be a challenge; and transportation can be problematic.

▶ *Assisted Living*: Assisted living provides housing as well as supervision, personal care services, meals, and recreational activities. It is, however, expensive, generally elderly-focused, and lacking in medical supervision and oversight.

▶ *Nursing Home Care*: Nursing homes provide 24-hour skilled nursing care for complex, unstable conditions. However, most are elderly-focused and may not provide programming appropriate for the younger resident with MS.

Family Finances

WHILE MANY FAMILIES find it difficult and stressful to discuss their finances and financial management strategies, these discussions are extremely important—and helpful—in the context of planning for potential care needs. Long-term care services are expensive. It is important to know your income resources, assets, and all sources of financial support. It is also important to maximize your resources through tax benefits, trusts, asset protection, and Medicaid spend-down, if appropriate. Starting these discussions early provides time to do a financial assessment and strategize ways to maximize insurances, protect assets, and pursue eligibility for benefits and entitlements.

Developing a Plan

IF THE TIME does come when a family member with MS requires additional assistance and services, the next step is for the family to sit down together to develop a detailed plan of care. The plan should address all the needs that must be met and identify the family and community resources that could be put in place to address those needs.

The goal of most families is to keep their loved one at home and in the community for as long as possible, regardless of his or her physical status. Fortunately, in recent years, we have seen increasing government interest in supporting and funding home- and community-based services. There is finally an acknowledgement within the health and social service system that access to home health care, homemaker services, adult day programs, and respite care is imperative if families are to care for loved ones with chronic disease and disability at home.

There is no question, however, that the time can come when safety issues in the home, or the chronic care needs of the family member with MS can exceed family resources, and a residential option will need to be explored. For individuals who continue to be capable of self-management and who have the financial resources, assisted living is certainly one alternative. In addition to providing housing in a semi-independent setting, most assisted living facilities also provide supportive services (e.g., meals, emergency assistance, and some personal care). However, if clinical and medical needs exceed what either home or assisted residential care can provide, then it becomes a priority to find a skilled nursing facility that is equipped to address the unique and complex needs of a person with MS.

It is important for families to be aware of the continuum of options and to be able to evaluate the appropriateness of these services and settings for the person with MS. This is particularly challenging since many of these programs primarily serve the frail elderly, not younger people with MS and other adult-onset disability. Therefore, services need to be reviewed, not only in terms of availability and quality of care, but in terms of whether they can provide appropriate services for a younger, non-elderly population.

There are numerous questions that need to be asked by families as they explore and engage a network of services and support.

Meeting a person's needs at home raises questions such as the following:

> What kind of help is required? Are we talking about companionship, home upkeep, or personal hands-on care? Obviously, the level of skill needed for each of these services varies, and if one is purchasing any of these services from community agencies, the cost will vary as well. If a person only needs someone to run errands and vacuum the house, there is no need to be paying for a certified nurses aide.

> When is the help needed? Is it concentrated in the morning, in the evening, or throughout the day? Are there safety concerns that would require someone to be available at all times?

- How much help can family members and friends provide? How reliable can they be? What other demands are they dealing with in their lives? Can they do the tasks that are needed? Who will coordinate the schedule and the care? Can neighbors help? Are there church or fraternal organization volunteers that can help?
- If the decision is made to seek services from community agencies such as healthcare agencies, adult day programs, transportation services, or meals-on-wheels, who will make the contacts? Who will look into eligibility for subsidized services? If the family must pay, how will payment be arranged? Who will pay for what?
- If the decision is made to hire help privately, who will interview applicants? Where will the interviews take place? Who will check references? How will payment be arranged? Who will train a new employee? Who will learn about wage and benefit regulations?
- Who will explore options for home modifications, durable medical equipment, and technological devices that will optimize independence and necessitate less hands-on care?

If families are exploring assisted living options, the following questions should be considered?

- Can the person with MS maintain a fairly high level of independence? Can he or she manage dressing, grooming, feeding, and toileting relatively independently?
- Will the person with MS require on-going medical supervision and oversight? Is there 24-hour nursing staff on site?
- Is the person with MS capable of self-management and self-direction of care?
- Is assisted living a regulated industry in their state? What facilities are licensed?
- What regulations are in place in the state regarding admission criteria for assisted living? Can all these criteria be met? For example, many states require that residents be able to transfer independently.
- How accessible is the facility if wheeled mobility is used?

- Is there a non-elderly population in the facility, or a desire to individualize programming for a younger resident?
- Is there a willingness for staff to be trained in MS and its implications?
- Are there specific discharge criteria that could necessitate having to move out of the facility if functioning declined?
- Almost 95% of assisted living is paid on a private pay basis. Is the family able to pay the monthly fee that could range from $1800-$4500? What does this fee cover? What are defined as additional services for which additional fees will be charged? If the cost of assisted living is prohibitive, does the state have a Medicaid waiver program to pay for assisted living? What are the eligibility criteria?

In evaluating skilled nursing facilities, the following issues should be addressed:

- Is the facility's state license up to date? What is their record of complaints and deficiencies?
- What does the "Nursing Home Compare" section of the Center of Medicare and Medicaid Services website, www.medicare.gov , say about the facility in terms of number of residents, staff-resident ratios, inspection results, and survey data?
- Does the facility accept Medicaid? Who will clarify eligibility criteria? If paying privately, what financial resources will be available? Who will pay the monthly fee? Will there be additional costs?
- Are there younger residents in the facility? Do any of them have MS or other neuro-degenerative diseases? How much experience has the facility had with MS? Are they open to having staff receive special training in this area?
- How elderly-focused are the activities? Is there interest in incorporating activities appealing to a younger population in terms of music, community outings, intellectually stimulating games and discussion, computer access, etc.? What particular interests and activities does the person with MS most want to preserve?

- How handicapped accessible is the facility? Does it have ramps, handrails, accessible bathrooms, and lifts? Is the importance of wheeled mobility appreciated? Is there storage available for equipment? Does it have arrangements with vendors who can supply and repair wheelchairs and other durable medical equipment?
- What healthcare professionals are on staff—physicians, physical therapists, occupational therapists, social workers, etc?
- What preventive care is available, such as immunizations, cancer screenings, dental care, eye care, foot care, etc?
- How are direct care staff assigned? Do they rotate throughout the facility, or work on specific units?
- Is there individual climate control for residents' rooms?

These lists of questions are not intended to be all-inclusive or complete. Rather, they are meant to guide families as they anticipate decisions and seek relevant information about the appropriateness and quality of various services and programs. Each family's specific questions will be based on the particular clinical and support needs of the person with MS, as well as the issues and concerns of greatest importance to family members.

MS is a variable and frustrating disease. It puts tremendous pressure on families because there is no way of knowing what lies ahead. Perhaps the MS will have a stable course and life will be relatively uneventful. On the other hand, there may be downturns and detours that will be unsettling and require adjustments and alternative planning. The process of looking to the future, evaluating options, and planning accordingly is like purchasing an insurance policy. The coverage may never be needed. But if the time comes when it is necessary, what a relief to know that everything that could be done has been done, and that the family is prepared and ready to take control and move forward.

ADDITIONAL READINGS

National MS Society Publications
Redford T. A Guide for Caregivers.
Hiring Help at Home: The Basic Facts.
Harmon J. At Home with MS: Adapting Your Environment.

Nursing Home Care of Individuals with Multiple Sclerosis: Guidelines and Recommendations for Quality Care

Assisted Living for Individuals with Multiple Sclerosis: Guidelines and Recommendations

PUBLICATION AVAILABLE FROM THE NATIONAL MS SOCIETY

National Endowment for Financial Education *Adapting: Financial Planning for a Life with Multiple Sclerosis, 2003.*

GENERAL READINGS

Frankel D. Long-term care. In: Kalb R. (ed.) *Multiple Sclerosis: The Questions You Have; The Answers You Need* (3rd ed.) New York: Demos Medical Publishing, 2004.

Cooper L. Life planning. In: Kalb R, (ed.) *Multiple Sclerosis: The Questions You Have; The Answers You Need* (3rd ed.). New York: Demos Medical Publishing, 2004.

RECOMMENDED RESOURCES

Assisted Living Federation of America (ALFA) (Tel: 703-691-8100; Internet: www.alfa.org).

Centers for Medicare and Medicaid Services (CMS) (Tel: 800-638-6833; Internet: www.cms.gov).

National Association for Home Care (Tel: 202-547-7424; Internet: www.nahc.org).

National Association of Professional Geriatric Care Managers (Tel: 520-881-8008; Internet: www.caremanager.org).

National Council on Aging (Tel: 202-479-1200; Internet: www.ncoa.org).

National Family Caregivers Association (Tel: 800-896-3650; Internet: www.nfcacares.org).

Social Security Administration (800-772-1213; Internet: www.medicare.gov).

Well Spouse Foundation (Tel: 800-838-0879; Internet: www.wellspouse.org).

11

General Health and Well-Being

Kathy Birk, M.D.
Elizabeth H Morrison, M.D., MSEd

Introduction

IT OFTEN HAPPENS that a person with MS meets an old friend who asks the usual question, "How are you?" The initial response from those who have a chronic illness may be, "Oh, not bad," or "Hanging in there," or "Hoping for the cure that will make my life better." While there is nothing wrong with these responses, individuals with MS can also choose to affirm their wellness without denying their illness. The eminent sociologist Arthur Frank writes that illness and wellness occupy two different continua; individuals with chronic conditions can therefore experience illness and wellness at the same time. Now is the time for people with MS, whether they use a wheelchair or scooter, are able-bodied with significant sensory symptoms or overwhelming fatigue, or have any of the other possible manifestations of MS, to respond "I am well." The goal is to embrace a philosophy of wellness while still honoring one's own life challenges.

General wellness relies on more than well-functioning myelin. In fact, a very wise physician, Sir William Osler, said, "If you develop a chronic illness and take the best possible care of it, you will live a longer and healthier life than those who do not have that advantage." Taking the best possible care of MS means more than treating the disease and its symptoms. It also means protecting one's general well being by adhering to *all* of the general preventive care guidelines for good health. People who have MS are certainly not immune to other medical problems, such as cardiac disease or cancer. They should embrace the kinds of preventive health care that goes beyond what is demanded by their MS. Family members of people with MS also need to take care of their own health.

Over the course of years living with the disease, people who have MS (and their doctors) have a tendency to focus on MS management to the exclusion of other significant health and wellness concerns. This chapter's goal is to remind all of us that having MS does not "protect" a person from developing other medical problems, and that various symptoms can be caused by issues other than MS. Healthy living and preventive care are just as important for people who have MS as they are for every other member of the family.

Making a Commitment to Wellness

MS CAN ROB people of significant control over some very basic elements of physical function and create uncertainty about the future degree of disability. Given that this is so, how can an individual maximize his or her feelings of control and strive to fulfill personal goals? Although the approved disease-modifying medications are helping to alter the course of the disease, the person with MS still needs to make a personal commitment to wellness. A particularly effective approach is for families affected by MS to work on wellness together.

Why, other than physical limitations, does health maintenance remain a low priority for so many people? "I don't have time" is the most common response. What is needed requires only a few hours in each person's week. (See Table 11.1)

The earlier such a routine becomes a part of your life, the better off you are. Here are some specific recommendations for making the best use of this relatively small weekly time commitment:

TABLE 11.1

RECOMMENDATIONS FOR WEEKLY HEALTH-PROMOTION BEHAVIORS

▶ Engage in 30 minutes of moderate-intensity exercise five times a week.

▶ Maintain a healthy body weight.

▶ Avoid smoking and recreational drug use, and use caution if you drink any alcohol, particularly if you have problems with walking or balance.

▶ Schedule an annual health maintenance visit with your primary care provider and follow up with needed testing, such as screening for high blood pressure, diabetes, elevated cholesterol, colon cancer, dental disease, breast and cervical cancer (for women), and testicular cancer (for men).

▶ Take a daily multivitamin and mineral supplement, and include at least 1000 mg of calcium in your diet every day (1500 mg for women after menopause or for any man or woman whose mobility or capacity for weight-bearing exercise is limited).

▶ Make time for safety practices in your daily life, including seat belts, violence prevention, and condoms if you are at risk for sexually transmitted diseases.

Exercise

REGULAR AEROBIC EXERCISE and strength training decrease the risk of cardiovascular disease, promote bone health, and improve overall quality of life. For these reasons, the Surgeon General recommends that all Americans strive to maintain a regular exercise program. Exercise is especially helpful in MS. A number of studies have found that exercise for people with MS provides many benefits, including improved fitness, muscle strength, and quality of life. Participants in some studies also had less disability, depression, pain, and fatigue.

Your physician can help you identify which type of exercise program would be most beneficial for you and which, if any, need to be avoided in order to protect certain muscle groups or reduce the risk of injury or over-exertion. An exercise "prescription" will often include a warm-up period with stretching, aerobic exercise that gives you a mild workout without making you short of breath, strengthening exercises, and a cool-down period. Your chapter of the National Multiple Sclerosis Society can steer you toward safe, supervised exercise programs. Your choice of exercise may be as simple as walking alone or with a group (even at malls) or taking a yoga class.

Protecting Your Heart

HEART DISEASE IS the leading cause of death for men and women in the United States. This is a fact that should invite everyone to:

- ▶ Not smoke.
- ▶ Maintain a healthy cholesterol level (usually, less than 200 for the total cholesterol and above 45 for the "good" HDL cholesterol).
- ▶ Make exercise a regular part of your life.
- ▶ Maintain an appropriate body weight, avoiding obesity.
- ▶ Follow your doctor's recommended schedule for regular health screening, which includes getting checked periodically for such conditions as high blood pressure, diabetes, and obesity.
- ▶ If you are over age 40, ask your doctor whether you should take a daily baby aspirin to prevent heart disease and stroke.

While prevention is the best policy, early detection is also important. MS could affect how a person experiences early warning signs of a heart attack or stroke, so it is important to remain vigilant for unusual symptoms. Stroke symptoms (e.g., visual changes or weakness), are easy to confuse with MS symptoms. Even without MS, women having heart attacks may not necessarily feel "classic" chest pain, but instead may experience nausea or shortness of breath. When in doubt, seek medical attention right away.

Nutrition

OBESITY IS A growing problem in this country, and efforts to maintain a healthy weight may be even more challenging for those who are less mobile. The following Dietary Guidelines for Americans have been published by the U.S. Department of Agriculture:

- ▶ Eat a variety of healthy foods.
- ▶ Balance the food you eat with physical activity to maintain or lower your weight.
- ▶ Choose a diet that contains plenty of grains, vegetables, and fruits.
- ▶ Limit your intake of fat (especially saturated fat) and cholesterol.
- ▶ Choose a diet that is moderate in sugar (including corn syrup) and salt (sodium).
- ▶ If you drink alcoholic beverages, do so in moderation.

People with MS who have balance, mobility, or cognitive problems might want to consider eliminating alcohol completely since the effects of alcohol can increase them. Regular dental care maintains healthier teeth, which will also promote good nutrition.

Fortunately, the information necessary to help us comply with these recommendations is now readily available. The newly-revised food guide pyramid (available at MyPyramid.gov) is designed to help you choose the foods and amounts that are right for you. Seeking advice from a nutritionist may be a reasonable step to take, along with purchasing one of the many books available about healthful eating. However you choose to pursue healthy nutrition, the following elements in your diet need careful attention:

Sodium. The salt in our diet comes not only from the saltshaker on the table, but also from almost all processed foods (e.g., canned soups and frozen dinners). It is important to pay attention to the labels on packaged foods in order to consume less than 2400 mg of sodium a day.

Calcium. Most people consume too little of this essential mineral. Some individuals, including women at or near menopause, and women or men whose mobility is restricted or who use steroids, need to be especially careful to obtain appropriate amounts of calcium in order to maintain healthy bones. Individuals who rely primarily on a scooter or wheelchair for mobility are particularly prone to bone loss. Smoking or a family history of osteoporosis are also reasons to increase calcium intake. The Revised Daily Elemental Calcium Requirements published by the National Institutes of Health include:

- ▶ 1000 mg per day for adults 25 to 65 years old.
- ▶ 1500 mg per day for postmenopausal women.

For the best absorption of calcium, it is important to obtain 400 international units (IU) of vitamin D from the foods you eat or from a dietary supplement. Dairy products (especially milk) often include vitamin D. Spending a brief time in the sun each day can also help.

Skim milk or any other low-fat dairy products such as yogurt or reduced-fat cheese are good dietary sources of calcium, as are other foods specially fortified with extra calcium (e.g., certain cereals and juices). Since it is difficult to obtain adequate calcium from diet alone, adults should also consider calcium supplements. Calcium carbonate, the most readily absorbed form of calcium, is available in a variety of supplement forms. Although many calcium supplements contain small amounts of lead, the benefits of calcium for most adults, especially adults with MS, are believed to outweigh any risk from lead. Some calcium citrate supplements contain less lead but are also more difficult for the body to absorb. A compromise would be to look for a supplement that is labeled "lead-free." Because calcium supplements do not typically include vitamin D, adding a multivitamin that contains vitamin D will help your body process the calcium.

In summary, a diet that is guided by the food pyramid and includes sufficient grains for fiber, along with lots of fresh fruits and vegetables, fat-free or low-fat dairy products, and supplements of calcium with vitamin D can help control weight and avoid osteoporosis. This relatively simple diet will also help prevent constipation, heart disease, and some cancers.

Preventive Health Care

IN ADDITION TO proper diet and exercise, periodic health appraisals and screening tests are essential. Regular evaluations should occur once a year. Health maintenance evaluations should include a health history, physical examination, and laboratory tests depending on age and history. Beyond this basic, general testing, certain special screening tests should be done at regular intervals that depend on the person's age:

▶ Breast or testicular examination done by a healthcare provider
▶ Blood testing for cholesterol
▶ Rectal examination for men and women after age 40 years
▶ Stool blood examination and other colon cancer testing for men and women after age 50 years, or if symptoms appear
▶ Pap smear for women of reproductive age, usually once a year
▶ Annual mammogram for women after age 40-50 years
▶ For those with MS, blood testing for thyroid problems.

Those with greater physical disability may worry that Pap tests, colon cancer screening, or mammography will be difficult to obtain. Many communities now offer accessible facilities for preventive health examinations. Some medical offices have special examination tables that lower to the floor. For pelvic examinations, the practitioner can use other adaptive equipment or techniques to increase comfort and avoid fatigue. It is certainly worthwhile to tell your practitioner in advance if you have any special needs.

People who have a chronic illness or disability may also have a tendency to neglect their dental health. Guidelines for accessing optimal dental care are available from the National MS Society (see Additional Reading p. 193).

Immunizations

ALTHOUGH WE MAY think of immunizations as interventions for children, even adults sometimes need immunizations to protect their health. The Centers for Disease Control and Prevention recommend these shots for adults:

- Tetanus and diphtheria (Td) booster every 10 years
- Annual influenza immunization (flu shot) if you are over 50 or if you have certain medical indications (Most MS Specialist neurologists recommend a yearly flu shot for their patients.)
- Pneumococcal (pneumonia) immunization if you are over age 65
- Varicella (chicken pox) immunization if you have not had the chicken pox.

With or without MS, you may also need other immunizations, depending on your medical history and on whether you plan to travel abroad.

Safety Issues

THERE ARE MANY things you and your family can do to make your daily lives safer and healthier. Important safety measures include:

- Wearing seat belts every time you drive or ride in a motor vehicle.
- Using condoms to prevent sexually transmitted diseases if you are sexually active.
- Avoiding excessive sun exposure and applying protective sunscreen when you will be in the sun.
- Keeping no firearms in the house, or at least keeping them securely locked.
- Avoiding tobacco and drugs, and drinking alcohol in moderation if at all.
- Protecting yourself and others from domestic violence.

The media publicize reports of abuse against women, children and even elders. Many Americans do not realize, however, that younger adults with disabilities can also be abused or neglected in the home. If you are concerned about possible abuse or neglect in any form, contact your local protective services agency or police department. There are also community resources available to help with alcohol and drug problems. Smokers who wish to quit can ask their doctors about new medications and behavioral strategies, or dial 1-800-NO-BUTTS.

Stress Management

GOOD PREVENTIVE HEALTH care includes finding comfortable and effective ways to manage the stresses of everyday life. Stress management can take a variety of forms; the primary goal should be to identify activities or techniques that you enjoy enough to continue doing on a regular basis. While one person may unwind by attending a support group or an exercise class, another may read, listen to music, or write in a journal. Regular recreational activities, such as playing cards, going to the movies, or gathering with friends for dinner are also important strategies for easing the tensions of daily living. Keep in mind that although some people need time alone in order to relax and unwind, others seek group activities or social interaction as a way to relieve stress.

People who find themselves feeling overwhelmed and out of control of the stresses in their lives should not hesitate to consult a psychotherapist. A mental health professional can help you identify the sources of stress in your life as well as effective management strategies. A consultation may be all you need to get started on your own stress management approach.

Midlife and Menopause in Women

BECAUSE THE AVERAGE life expectancy for women is now more than 80 years, women can expect to spend at least one-third of their lives after menopause. In fact, one-third of the women in the United States have been through "the change." Learning what to expect from these hormonal and age-related changes is vital, especially for those who have MS, because certain peri-menopausal symptoms may be confused with a worsening of the disease. Hormones have indeed been found to have some impact on MS. This impact is greatest during and after pregnancy, as is described in Chapter 5. In addition, the symptoms of MS may increase at ovulation (midway through the menstrual cycle) when body temperature rises slightly and the estrogen level is at its peak. During the next 2 weeks until the period occurs, the temperature remains slightly elevated while the estrogen level gradually declines.

Estrogen, which declines during menopause, plays a major role in the health of the body, especially of the bones and heart. It is because of estrogen that women are much less likely than men to begin having heart attacks before the age of 60. When estrogen levels decline, bone density or thickness likewise decreases. Although bone density can begin to decline long before midlife, a truly dramatic decline begins at menopause. This trend is most often reflected in women's increased fracture risk (especially of the hip, wrist, and spine) after age 60. Women should, therefore, make every effort to arrive at menopause with the maximum bone density possible. Promoting healthy bones is best accomplished with weight-bearing exercise and calcium intake starting in childhood and continuing through the teens and twenties, when the body's maximum bone mass is developing. Once this bone density has been established, it needs to be maintained in the thirties, forties, and thereafter. (See the "Nutrition" section earlier in this chapter for a detailed discussion of calcium requirements.)

Adults with MS or other risk factors for osteoporosis (thinning of the bones leading to risk of fractures) should also have special screening tests done. While osteoporosis is common in women after menopause, especially if they are thin and of Caucasian or Asian ancestry, it can also occur in men and women of any age who use steroids or who have limited mobility. It is now possible to determine a person's bone density using a DEXA® (dual energy X-ray absorptiometry) scan, which is a simple, painless, and safe test that predicts a person's relative fracture risk based on a computer-generated graph. There are also other methods of osteoporosis screening that your healthcare provider may recommend. Women or men who have osteoporosis may be prescribed a medication such as alendronate, which can increase bone density and help prevent fractures. As always, exercise and calcium must also be a part of the treatment.

Because menopause is the beginning of the rest of a woman's (long) life, the recommendations for preventive health care continue to apply during midlife and beyond. In general, physical exercise and a low-fat diet that includes the recommended 25–35 grams of daily fiber and adequate calcium continue to be essential to promote wellness. Routine preventive testing should include cholesterol screening, mammograms, Pap testing for cervical cancer, and screening for diseases such as colon cancer, high blood pressure, and diabetes.

Hormone replacement therapy is an important issue that all women of menopausal age need to consider. In years past, health practitioners routinely recommended hormone replacement for postmenopausal women because preliminary data suggested that estrogen supplements would decrease women's risk of heart attacks, strokes, cognitive problems, osteoporosis, and fractures. These preliminary studies were mostly of an observational variety, which could only suggest health benefits without truly proving them.

Proof depended on nationwide trials that would yield more definitive data by randomly assigning women to hormone replacement or to placebo medications, tracking outcomes over multiple years. When these long-term trials began to yield results, they showed that hormone replacement did *not* provide the expected preventive benefits. Not only did estrogen and progestin not prevent heart attacks, they indeed seemed to cause them. The research also found that postmenopausal hormone replacement therapy increased the risk of breast cancer. Even though the studies found that hormone replacement prevented osteoporosis and fractures, relatively few physicians believe this benefit outweighs the increased risks of heart disease and breast cancer, especially since there are safe and effective treatments available for osteoporosis.

There are good reasons that some women may choose to use estrogen and progestin after menopause. Women bothered by hot flushes or other menopausal symptoms, for instance, might discuss with their physicians whether they should try hormone replacement for a period of time. Vaginal dryness or similar symptoms that may be MS-related, however, will not improve with hormone therapy. A woman's use of estrogen and progestin for short-term relief of menopausal symptoms should depend on discussions with her practitioner about the potential benefits and risks given her particular medical history, family history, and symptoms. Most physicians no longer recommend long-term use of hormone replacement therapy for the goal of preventing heart disease, osteoporosis or other medical problems.

Many over-the-counter remedies can alleviate perimenopausal symptoms. Vaginal moisturizers (KY Jelly®, Astroglide®, Replens®, and others) can increase comfort. Vitamin E (400 IU per day) has long been thought to reduce hot flashes. Soy products (soy milk, tofu) can result in healthier hearts and bones and can decrease hot flashes. Natural and health food stores encourage the use of dong quai, ginseng, black cohosh, wild yam root, and other products. Be careful, however, because acceptable studies are only now under way to assess the risk-benefit ratio of many complementary and alternative therapies.

We all want to make the right decisions about our health, knowing we will be living with them for a lifetime. Unfortunately, women (and men) are faced with decisions for which there are no guarantees and may be no obvious right answers. Medical recommendations vary from doctor to doctor and from study to study. The important thing is to be well informed, to discuss the issues thoroughly with your doctor, and to re-evaluate your choices as new research becomes available.

Conclusions

THIS CHAPTER HAS described some of the important health and wellness concerns of individuals with MS and their family members. Careful attention to health-promoting behaviors will make you an active participant in the teamwork that is required for you to enjoy the highest possible quality of life and be able to respond, "I am well, thank you" to all who inquire. It is important to make sure that the practitioners with whom you are working are sensitive to these concerns and attentive to problems other than those directly related to MS.

Although this discussion of general wellness has highlighted the health of the person who has MS, the same recommendations hold true for family members and friends. It is not only people who have a chronic illness who tend to forget preventive health care measures. Caregivers of very disabled individuals may find themselves so involved with MS-related demands that they neglect their own health or withdraw from healthy and relaxing activities that the person with MS can no longer share. On the other hand, people with MS who are able and willing to strive for wellness may find themselves becoming role models who inspire those around them. Please see Chapter 8 for a discussion of the experience of families and friends of people with MS. Whatever your own personal and family situation, it is essential to pay attention to your own health and well being. To the extent that everyone can adopt this approach, life's stresses—including the stresses of MS—will become smaller factors in what should be a happier and healthier family life.

ADDITIONAL READINGS

National MS Society Publications
    (available by calling 1-800-FIGHT-MS (1-800-344-4867) or
    online at http://www.nationalmssociety.org/library.asp)
Choosing the Right Health-Care Provider
Clear Thinking about Alternative Therapies
Dental Health: The Basic Facts
Exercise as Part of Everyday Life
Food for Thought: MS and Nutrition
Managing MS Through Rehabilitation
Multiple Sclerosis and Your Emotions
Preventive Care Recommendations for Adults with MS: The Basic Facts
Taming Stress in Multiple Sclerosis
Vitamins, Minerals, and Herbs in MS: An Introduction

GENERAL READINGS

Frank AW. The Wounded Storyteller: Body, Illness, and Ethics. Chicago: University of Chicago Press, 1995.

Kraft GH, Catanzaro M. *Living with Multiple Sclerosis: A Wellness Approach* (2nd ed.). New York: Demos Medical Publishing, 2000).

Spero D. *The Art of Getting Well: A Five-Step Plan for Maximizing Health When You Have a Chronic Illness.* Alameda, CA: Hunter House, 2002. ordering@hunterhouse.com

RECOMMENDED RESOURCES (INTERNET)

College of American Pathologists—Offers a free service (www. MyHealthTest Reminder.com) that sends e-mail reminders for mammograms, Pap tests, and screening for diabetes, cholesterol, and colon cancer.

Centers for Disease Control (CDC) and Prevention: Immunization recommendations for adults available online at http:// www.cdc.gov/nip/recs/adult-schedule.htm.

12

Life Planning: Financial and Legal Considerations for Families Living with MS

Laura D. Cooper, JD

E FFECTIVE LIFE PLANNING involves taking steps now to protect yourself and your family in the future. Although relatively few people who have multiple sclerosis (MS) become incapacitated enough to require long-term care, there is no way to predict with any certainty who will become severely disabled and who will not. Therefore, the optimal strategy is to implement plans now that will ensure your family's financial security regardless of the ultimate severity of the disease. It goes without saying that disability is a circumstance that no one would opt for. When it does occur, the key to a rich, fulfilling life, regardless of disability level, lies in planning.

The subject of life planning is one that most people find distressing. No one particularly enjoys thinking about potential problems or losses. However, engaging in the process of long-range planning and problem-solving will enable you to feel secure about your family's well-being, regardless of what the future brings. This chapter highlights the principal components in the planning process. Because each family's situation is unique, and the complex laws pertaining to these issues vary considerably from state to state, the information provided here should in no way be considered comprehensive. You are well advised to consult an elder law attorney who specializes in disability-related law and/or a certified financial planner to discuss your family's particular needs. Your chapter of the National Multiple Sclerosis Society can recommend an appropriate professional in your area.

Selecting Planning Professionals to Assist You

A STRONG WORD of caution must be offered here about selecting planning professionals to assist you. Only a few certified financial planners have the experience and expertise necessary to construct a rational and workable financial plan in the face of potentially career-shortening disability or illness. That is because most financial planners are, in fact, wealth planners, whose expertise is *not* designed for middle-class clients. Thus, most financial planners are *not* experts in assisting *average* or *middle-class* people to make sound financial decisions and deploying their resources most effectively.[1]

This is particularly important to keep in mind when an individual needs to construct a sound financial plan in the face of potentially devastating illness or disability. Most typical planning strategies are inadequate in this situation; individuals who mistakenly rely on "traditional wisdom" are likely to face serious— but otherwise avoidable—financial disasters.[2] As a consequence, *it is critical that you exercise great caution when selecting financial experts or advice and screen for specific expertise in the area of disability planning.*

Some key points include:

[1] For example, the typical planner's advice to have about 6 months of expenses available in liquid assets in case of emergency is pitifully unrealistic advice for any person who must survive the waiting period for a Social Security Disability claim. A more realistic time period for such "emergency" planning is about two years, and a good middle-class financial plan would take account of that fact and assist the client to take reasonable steps to prepare for that situation.

[2] For example, most financial planners encourage their clients to rely heavily on employer-sponsored welfare benefits (such as health and disability benefits) because of their favored tax status. Unfortunately, employer-sponsored benefits have very limited and inferior legal remedies—which encourages more recalcitrant insurer behavior than other forms of coverage. In addition, employer-sponsored benefits are noncontinuous as a matter of law and that is the reason many people who become too ill to work end up losing their health benefits. Individuals who do not rely completely upon employer-sponsored health benefits, on the other hand, have

- A well-versed financial advisor assisting an individual with a potentially career-shortening disability will place a great deal of emphasis on the "risk" or insurance plan, and will pay particular attention to *continuity of coverage* problems that may arise with employer-sponsored coverage that disappears with the termination of employment.
- If the advice offered is simplistic, or relies solely on "traditional" insurance or savings strategies, that advice may well be inadequate to assist people with potentially career-shortening illnesses to reach specific financial objectives.

What is Life Planning?

IN ITS MOST basic form, life planning is a process that encourages you to think about what you want in life (to set life goals), and to formulate a workable plan for ensuring that you are able to achieve those goals. The most important aspect of the plan is that it should be well executed and comprehensive. A well-developed plan addresses all contingencies so that the possibility of its not being implemented approaches zero. In other words, a comprehensive plan should leave virtually nothing to chance. It should include many different aspects of formal individual planning, including financial, estate, and vocational plans. The planning process requires a consideration of everything that is important to the individual for whom the plan is being developed.

The life-planning process takes on special significance for persons with severe disabilities because their social and financial futures are so tenuous. Contrary to popular myth, it is not only the wealthy who must plan. The fewer resources you have, the *more*

---

additional sources of coverage when they must leave work. Despite this potentially fatal flaw in a financial plan that is based solely on employer-sponsored benefits, it is difficult to find any mainstream financial planning advice that does not encourage or assume reliance upon employer-sponsored health benefits. Nor is the cost of dual coverage prohibitive if a client is steered to the right sources for coverage. For example, a good catastrophic excess major medical policy that overlaps an employer plan and provides excellent benefits for serious illness can cost as little as $10 per month for a young single person, and only a few hundred dollars per year for an entire family, and is sometimes available on a guaranteed issue basis.

important it is that you plan wisely in order to deploy your scarce resources in the most efficient and effective manner possible. Similarly, the greater the potential medical or vocational liabilities you may have, the more you need to ensure that you are adequately prepared for the expenses of illness, disability, or unemployment.

The Elements of Life Planning

WHERE SHOULD YOU begin? Before diving right in, you should become familiar with some key concepts. In the face of disability or illness, the most important aspects of planning will involve anticipating your financial risks (as opposed to growing assets, for example). The first principle of risk planning is that you must plan for the *worst* scenario. Otherwise, if the worst occurs, you will likely be unprepared for its potentially devastating effects. If, by planning in advance for them, you are prepared to meet the most difficult challenges head on, you will avoid having to cope with devastating financial loss at precisely the time when you are least emotionally equipped to do so.

In reality, every person has a life plan. The plan may simply be to take things as they come, to live from paycheck to paycheck, and to presume, therefore, that one will not become old, sick, or disabled. The life-planning process described in this chapter is, quite simply, a concerted effort to avoid such a non-approach. Nor is it too late to begin planning *after* the diagnosis. Some form of planning, whenever it occurs, is always better than having no specific agenda whatsoever.

Essentially, the life-planning process is designed to help a person reduce risk by (1) thinking through all possible contingencies, and (2) developing appropriate strategies to prevent life events from dictating catastrophic outcomes based on chance. The process includes four major types of planning:

- ▶ Life circumstances planning, or planning personal needs in major areas of life
- ▶ Planning for advocacy and directives by choosing professional and personal representatives or guardians in advance, as well as formulating advance directives

▶ Planning and implementing an ample financial portfolio or set of financial strategies designed to provide a financial portfolio, given the life goals that you have set, including provisions for adequate insurance against large financial risks

▶ Preparing estate plans

A fifth activity includes organizing all critical records into a health records file in order to permit continuity of administration of affairs throughout any period of disability, as well as after death. Regulations and penalties for medical providers who share medical information have become daunting. Such regulations also provide incentives for medical providers to dispose of older medical records. As a consequence, you may not be able to rely on your medical providers to keep a complete, long-term medical record for you. With the complexities of the information age, it is now in *each individual's own interest* to keep a thorough record of his or her own health history. You would be well advised, therefore, to create and maintain a complete, private medical record for yourself, including copies of imaging reports, lab reports, and any other record critical to your own long-term healthcare.

Perhaps the *most important* aspect of the life plan will be a comprehensive *insurance plan* (see pp. 208-204). The traditional financial model in the United States assumes that an individual will begin working as a young adult and continue—essentially uninterrupted—until retirement age. MS can dramatically alter that model in several fundamental ways: the disease could cause your work life to be substantially shortened, thereby reducing the number of years in which you are able to accrue resources; the disease could also cause you to start drawing upon your savings at a premature age, and also cause you to have to draw upon those savings for a longer time than the typical retirement period; additionally, the disease could easily *increase your overall expenses*.

It is unrealistic to think that a typical middle-class person will be able to save sufficient resources to allow him or her to retire prematurely, stay retired longer, and have higher overall health-related expenses for any length of time in retirement. Thus, the *most* critical element of the life plan will be construction of the risk or insurance plan as part of the financial plan. In fact, the insurance plan may drive all of the other components of the life plan; if there is a *shortage* of life, health, or disability coverage, the possible resulting limited financial resources if disability were to intrude could require a fundamental retooling of the entire life plan, including altering of life goals.

Life Circumstances Planning

TRADITIONALLY, LIFE CIRCUMSTANCES planning includes planning for housing, living arrangements, education, employment, transportation, long-term services, and other social objectives. Life circumstances planning is the most important early step because it will determine the overall setting in which the life plan will be implemented. For example, choosing to live in an isolated, rural area will certainly challenge efforts to obtain necessary personal services and transportation. Choosing any type of housing that has architectural barriers may itself impede independence and accentuate disability. On the other hand, accessible housing on reliable public transportation lines in a metropolitan area may be difficult to find as well as expensive.

Location and housing type will, in turn, dictate the price and availability of various forms of long-term services, as well as educational and employment opportunities. Moreover, the cost of almost every element of the life plan will be strongly influenced by the location and type of residence you select. The ideal housing location will allow you to take advantage of educational, community, and employment opportunities that meet your personal goals, and afford you access to all the long-term services you need (and can afford) in case of severe illness or disability.

Perhaps the best way to perform this life circumstances planning is to construct a letter of intent. This informal document is a way to communicate important information about yourself to individuals who might provide care for you or exercise judgment on your behalf in the future. A letter of intent encourages you to sit down and think about what you want for yourself. Although it is not legally binding, a letter of intent is a useful document. It should include information about you, your family members, other relationships, advocates, medical history and care, housing, religious values, other systems of values, final arrangements, education, daily living skills, work life, government or private benefits available, hobbies and interests, and anything else that comprises an important personal life factor.

The letter of intent serves as the core of the life circumstances planning process, and provides important information regarding necessary or available types and amounts of financial resources for both the financial and estate planning processes. Before a person with a disability begins working up a financial or estate plan, he or she is well advised to complete a thorough life circumstances plan and make decisions about housing, transportation, education, and other social circumstances.

Planning For Advocacy And Directives

BECAUSE THE PLANNING process requires preparation for the worst-case scenario, a person with a disability must squarely face the possibility of catastrophic long-term illness and disability. It is this possibility that requires consideration of the issue of legal incompetence.

Every competent adult has the legal right to make decisions about his or her own medical care, including the decision to accept or refuse that care. Sometimes illness interferes with a person's ability to exercise that legal right. This occurs, for example, when a person becomes too cognitively impaired to make competent decisions. As a result, the person who is judged legally incompetent can no longer carry out his or her personal wishes. Unfortunately, this may occur at precisely the moment when those wishes would need to be followed because of the effects of illness. Under these circumstances, the person does not actually lose the right to make a decision; rather, the ability to carry out those wishes is lost due to legal incapacity to make the relevant decisions. To make matters even more difficult, healthcare providers need not abide by the decisions of an individual who has been judged legally incompetent if those decisions conflict with the healthcare provider's own judgment.

The way to enforce your wishes about medical care decisions, even in the event that you become legally incompetent to make those decisions, is to make them *ahead of time* and place them in a set of legally enforceable "advance directives."[3] Doing so preserves your legal ability to carry out your wishes as stated in the advance directive, even after you are incapacitated. If you have a legally enforceable advance directive, healthcare providers must be directed by those wishes whether or not they agree with them.

⊙ Advance Directives

ADVANCE DIRECTIVES ARE written documents in which competent persons state their anticipated medical decisions for the future. Directives can be communicated in one of two ways: (1) by making express written directives to healthcare providers, as in a *living will*, or (2) by designating another person who knows and would be sympathetic to your desires when the time for decision-making arrived, if you were too incapacitated to make your wishes known. This second form of advance directive is known as a *healthcare proxy* or *power of attorney for healthcare decision-making*.

Although the living will and healthcare proxy are both advance directives, many standardized forms for directives only incorporate one of these two types (usually only a limited living will). No matter which standardized form you may be offered, a complete set of advance directives should include both a living will *and* a healthcare proxy.

The basic distinction between a living will and a healthcare proxy is the type of directive involved. A living will establishes certain treatment guidelines that are to be followed in the future. A healthcare proxy does not establish treatment guidelines directly. Rather, it appoints a trusted person to act as your agent (proxy) in making healthcare decisions for you if you have become too incapacitated to make them yourself. A healthcare proxy can incorporate provisions of a living will by requiring that the proxy follow any directives stated in a separate living will, or by incorporating the living will directly into the healthcare proxy (in which case, the authority of the chosen proxy would be limited by the living will conditions stated in the

3 Advance directive requirements vary greatly from state to state.

healthcare proxy). Because it is almost impossible to predict all circumstances that might arise during any future illness, it would be difficult to place all advance directives in a living will. A healthcare proxy in conjunction with a living will is necessary to safeguard your right to self-determination. Consequently, a good set of advance directives will include both a living will and a healthcare proxy.

If you become incapacitated without leaving any specific directives, your family members will generally be considered suitable substitute decision-makers. In theory, most courts agree that family members are the appropriate decision-makers, even in the absence of a proxy. In practice, however, family member decisions that are made without an enforceable healthcare proxy are not followed by healthcare providers if the providers question the good faith of the family members or strongly disagree with the medical decision. On the other hand, if an enforceable healthcare proxy specifically appoints the family member as proxy, healthcare providers must treat the decisions made by your proxy as if you had made them yourself. They would not be able to deviate from those decisions even if they happened to disagree with them. Advance directives that specifically appoint a proxy therefore provide protection against healthcare providers who would be hesitant to follow your values (as understood by your proxy) when you are incapacitated. Thus, healthcare proxies are critical devices for people who hold any values that differ substantially from those of the healthcare community.

⊙ A Proxy vs. a Surrogate

IT IS ON this issue that an important legal distinction must be made between a *proxy* and a *surrogate*. A proxy implies that a person is designated in an advance directive, and is therefore someone appointed directly by the incapacitated patient. A surrogate is someone who is legally appointed outside of an advance directive. For example, if no valid healthcare proxy exists, a surrogate may be appointed to make decisions for the incapacitated patient. A family member appointed without an enforceable advance directive is a surrogate. This surrogate may become empowered either by a legal relationship that automatically gives rise to the right to make surrogate decisions (such as a family member) or by appointment as guardian by a court.

The extent to which a decision-maker can enforce decisions about the future care of a loved one will depend on whether the decision-maker was appointed by a healthcare proxy, in which case he or she is acting as proxy, or by some other process of law, in which case the person is legally understood to be a surrogate decision-maker. That these two types of decision-makers are regarded differently can be seen most clearly in quality- of-life determinations (e.g., the decision to remove life support because the patient's quality of life has diminished below an acceptable level). Decisions by proxies are almost invariably followed with respect to quality-of-life decisions, in keeping with an individual's right of self-determination. However, decisions regarding quality of life made by surrogates are examined with close scrutiny to make sure that they conform to the incapacitated individual's desires or best interests. Again, the best way to ensure that your wishes are followed is to execute a complete set of advance directives.

Financial Planning

FINANCIAL PLANNING IS the methodical process of evaluating your total assets, liabilities, and future income potential, and then using that information to determine your best options for meeting future needs and wants. Plans should be made as soon as possible for the family members or friends who provide support, as well as the person who has MS. The plans should then be revised periodically or as new circumstances dictate. The planning process may include the assessment of a myriad of financial options, including insurance, annuities, pensions, home equity, and availability of government benefits. Certified financial planners and lawyers may be valuable in sorting through the options and identifying the possible legal and tax consequences of various choices and choice combinations.

The normal process of financial planning requires a sequential series of steps, including:

1. Determining your financial situation.
2. Setting goals.
3. Developing a plan.
4. Keeping simple records.
5. Making an informal budget.
6. Dealing with shortfalls, credit, and debt.
7. Reviewing your progress.

However, financial planning for families with members who have a disability is fundamentally different. Families with a member who has a disability that could become severe enough to require long-term services cannot normally be expected to earn enough to meet their own financial needs. Therefore, these families must develop alternative financial (and estate) plans that explicitly incorporate available government benefits. The resources required for long-term services are significantly lower if the person with a disability stays at home, has a disability that is less severe, and requires less assistance or supervision.

⊙ Safeguarding Your Family from Extraordinary Costs

IT IS IMPERATIVE in constructing a financial plan that you not only develop your assets, but also safeguard yourself and your family from the potential extraordinary costs of the unpredictable illness. When you are planning for such risk, the sensible approach is to assume that the worst will happen, and assess your position should that occur. Unfortunately, when we become ill, the messages we receive from some of our most trusted loved ones and advisors cause us to do just the opposite. Encouraged to be optimistic and hope for the best, we often neglect necessary planning. One should *never* plan for the best. Such a strategy is doomed to fail in all but the most ideal and infrequent circumstances. From a strict planning perspective, planning for the worst should adequately prepare you for whatever awful surprises may come your way, and leave you pleasantly surprised about how prepared you were if something less than the worst occurs.

For example, if you are the primary breadwinner in your family and you become disabled, you may jeopardize the continuation of your family's entire health insurance package. And, while you are laid up, you somehow have to provide income replacement for the time you are not working, including finding income supplements for additional expenses attributable to any disability you may incur. You may find it difficult or impossible at that point to increase your life insurance to provide ample financial security for your loved ones. And, even upon returning to work (assuming that you are able to do so, *and* that you are able to obtain adequate health insurance coverage from your employer), you may find that you are less productive than you were previously, and therefore less able to garner the same income. All of these possibilities are daunting, to say the least. If you planned for all of them, you might be able to salvage whatever lifestyle you had before your disability occurred. If you adequately planned for none or only some of them, a significant, long-term disability would markedly reduce the quality of life for yourself and your family members.

So, the question in this circumstance becomes how can someone deal with the financial risks attributable to ill health while maintaining an adequate earnings and savings strategy? The answer lies mostly in devising a strategy of protection planning for the risk of ill health. The object of protection planning is to find ways to reduce those risks, to make yourself and your loved ones as "bullet-proof" as possible, given whatever unpleasant surprises your MS or other health conditions might bring your way. You should have a protection plan for every member of your family, tailored for that family member's situation. Those plans will differ, depending on whether the disabled family member is the primary breadwinner, the supporting spouse or caretaker, or a child or other dependent. This is because the risks that matter, and the degree to which those risks jeopardize the accumulation of wealth, vary greatly, depending on the life circumstances of each individual. The important thing to remember is that even the lack of a formal protection plan *is* a protection plan, albeit an inadequate one that provides no insurance and no strategies for avoiding risks.

Regardless of actual costs, a family would need to be quite wealthy to rely exclusively on family dollars to finance the long-term expenses of the worst-case scenario. For this reason, it is absolutely essential for most families to create an estate plan that will ensure eligibility for government benefits. On the other hand, because government benefits are notoriously unreliable, a family should also make every effort to create an estate plan that relies on private dollars (including insurance dollars). Government benefits may only be awarded after a lengthy or costly legal battle; they are subject to legislative change (and so are difficult to plan for); and rules for eligibility may be narrowed or changed administratively as government policies or resources change. For example, a little-known provision of the Health Insurance Portability and Accountability Act of 1996 has made it a criminal offense (punishable by fines of up to $10,000 and jail sentences of up to 1 year) to apply for Medicaid during the disqualification period that follows any transfer of assets from one individual to another (for the purpose of achieving Medicaid eligibility). Thus, no application can be filed for Medicaid during the 36-month waiting period (60 months if a trust is involved) following the transfer of assets. This unfortunate provision, if allowed to remain, could seriously affect all elderly or seriously disabled individuals who look to Medicaid to cover the cost of nursing home services.

⊙ Government Benefits

WITH THOSE LIMITATIONS in mind, many people who have disabilities are eligible for benefits under one or more of several government programs. The design of the programs is generally to protect persons with disabilities by making sure that they have sufficient resources to provide the basic necessities of life, including food, clothing, shelter, and healthcare. The programs can be grouped into two categories: those based on financial need (i.e., Supplemental Security Income [SSI] and Medicaid), and those classified as social insurance programs (i.e., Social Security [SSDI] and Medicare). The former are available to individuals with disabilities who satisfy certain financial restrictions. The latter are potentially available regardless of financial assets, and are based on the premiums that have been paid into the program during the person's years of employment.

Unfortunately, the rules relating to these programs are very complicated and constantly in flux. Generally, however, in order to qualify for benefits as a person with a disability, a person must be considered to have a "disability" within the meaning of the particular government program. Under the rules of the Social Security Administration (SSA), which are used by most government agencies, a person is considered to have a disability if he or she is unable to engage in any *substantial gainful activity* by reason of any medically determinable physical or mental impairment that can be expected to result in death or that can be expected to last for a continuous period of at least 12 months. To SSA, a job constitutes "substantial gainful activity" if the pay is $500 or more per month, after deducting the cost of impairment-related work expenses. The rules are less strict for people who have visual impairments.

⊙ Insurance

BECAUSE GOVERNMENT CASH benefits are so unreliable and insubstantial, persons with disabilities are well advised to devise alternative methods for financing costs attributed to their own disabilities and illnesses. Given the potential enormity of liability, insurance is a logical alternative to direct financing of the potential liabilities.

Insurance takes the shape of a counterintuitive form of investment: you pay for something you hope you will never need to use. Because of the gloom inherent in these arrangements, some people hesitate to invest adequately in insurance coverage. This view, however, is risky wishful thinking unless you are very wealthy. Although you may never have enough dollars to pay for the potential devastating consequences of disability on your own, you can at least *minimize the risks* by insuring against them. Insurance is essentially a means of transferring financial risk to an outside party. Rather than risk all the consequences of disability, you instead pay a premium and transfer some of the risk to an insurance company.

As the probability increases of that risk coming to fruition, the cost to the insurance company increases correspondingly. Thus, the types of insurance that are most important to a disabled person are, unfortunately, precisely the types of insurance that become more difficult to obtain following the diagnosis of a significant medical condition (e.g., MS). The types of insurance that are directly affected by health conditions that the insurance industry considers serious enough to be "ratable" (i.e., to warrant a higher risk assessment) usually include:

- Life insurance.
- Health insurance.
- Disability insurance.
- Long-term care insurance.
- Disability-based insurance, such as:
  - Mortgage insurance.
  - Business overhead insurance.
  - Disability buy-sell insurance.
  - Key-person disability insurance.

Of course, the limited availability of insurance does not decrease the need for it. For example, life insurance has traditionally been purchased to take care of needs such as maintenance of dependents following the death of a breadwinner, payment of liabilities, payment for college expenses, and payment for extraordinary needs. These needs remain just as important—if not more important—for a disabled individual.

Life insurance.
Life insurance is essentially a pot of money available when we die. However, the life insurance *contract* itself has value even while the owner is still alive, because it represents *guaranteed payment in the future* of the proceeds of the policy. It is also possible, therefore, to view life insurance as a pot of money that is available *during life* for extraordinary needs, or as a substitute for some disability-related insurance products (e.g., mortgage insurance). For example, a person who knows that he or she is going to die can convert existing life insurance into current money. Unfortunately, life insurance cannot normally be used in this manner by persons with MS because it is not considered a terminal disease. However,

a well-spouse diagnosed with terminal cancer might want to make use of life insurance benefits in this way in order to generate needed funds more quickly. An attorney who specializes in elder law can provide information about the procedures involved and draw up the necessary contract with the *viatical* company offering this financial arrangement.

Another alternative is to use *whole life* insurance in place of *term life*, and then take out policy loans against the cash value of the whole life policy for extraordinary needs. Term life insurance (a form of life insurance that provides a fixed amount of money if the person dies within the stated term of the policy but has no additional investment value) is the insurance typically offered by employers. Whole life insurance (a form of investment that not only provides insurance but also accumulates cash value) is typically purchased privately by individuals. Assuming that you are able to obtain enough whole life insurance, you may be able to borrow enough against its value to defray the costs attributable to disability *during your lifetime.*

There are a number of ways that persons with a diagnosis of MS can obtain life insurance despite diagnosis. One way is to convert existing individual term life policies to whole life. Another way is to obtain as many group memberships as possible in associations that offer "guaranteed issue" life insurance (and then convert this to whole or universal life if offered). Also, a person with MS should accept as much employment-based life insurance as is available, and convert this insurance to whole life insurance if that option is available upon leaving employment.

Health insurance

Most consumers think of health insurance as one big package (that somebody else should pay for) that is designed to take care of all of their healthcare needs. In fact, most Americans make this mistake until they get sick and discover just how inadequate their benefits really are.

An insurance policy is simply a type of contract. You, the consumer, agree to pay an insurer a particular amount in exchange for which the insurer agrees to compensate you for particular expenses you incur in connection with certain health problems.

In that sense, health insurance can be thought of as a form of casualty insurance. Like other forms of casualty insurance, you need to pay attention to the types of problems that are covered, under what circumstances, and what exactly the insurer has agreed to pay when the casualty occurs.

The purpose of health insurance is to protect you and your family against the potentially catastrophic costs of medical expenses that can accompany a serious illness. Thus, in the overall scheme of things, health insurance is simply a means of protecting your other assets so that you will not have to drain them to pay for the expenses that can accompany a serious illness. Like other forms of insurance, health insurance is best purchased *before* a significant health issue arises. Policy-makers understandably discourage equality of coverage for both healthy and unhealthy individuals; if good health coverage were as readily available *after* an illness as *before* there would be little incentive for healthy people to shoulder any significant premium costs for good insurance, and the private insurance system would collapse.

Inadequacy of coverage for seriously ill or disabled individuals

Unfortunately, our government has encouraged employer-sponsorship of health insurance as the primary source of coverage in the private marketplace. Employers purchase health coverage that they believe will satisfy the needs of their employees. By marketing insurance to *employers* the coverage has been adapted to the demands of its purchasers. Thus, over time, more benefits have been provided for "working well" people, to the detriment of coverage for individuals who are seriously ill. Most traditional health plans now have inadequate coverage for seriously ill individuals, and in order to meet the increasing demands of the working well to whom the insurance is marketed, this trend is likely to continue. For example, many policies now include chiropractic and counseling benefits, but few policies still provide reasonable or adequate rehabilitation or therapy benefits, and those benefits that do exist are often prohibited for "maintenance" therapy (such as is required for MS). Similarly, coverage for durable medical equipment has been constrained over time, home healthcare coverage is becoming a rarity, and prescription formularies (the lists of medications that a company is willing to cover) are continuing to narrow. Most basic employer policies are simply inadequate for the needs of seriously ill individuals, and *anyone* who wants comprehensive health coverage *must* have a catastrophic major medical policy in addition to a basic employer plan.

Discontinuity of coverage

Adding to the dilemma of coverage deficits is the problem of *discontinuity*. Because our health insurance system is mostly based on *employer-sponsored* benefits, health benefits can only be considered as secure as the prospect of the employee's *continued employment*. In other words, the provider of employer-sponsored benefits is the *employer* and a break with the employer could eventually cause a break with the coverage. If your insurance is a benefit of your spouse or parent, the loss of that relationship (through divorce or death, for instance) could also deprive you of your critical health benefits.[4] Consequently, employer-sponsored health benefits lack the essential element of *continuity that we expect from every other insurance policy we own*, and a thorough insurance and financial plan should include specific strategies that can be implemented when or if employer-sponsored insurance becomes unavailable.

Steps to ensure continuity of health insurance

The first step in developing such a strategy is to know exactly what you will be entitled to get and when, regardless of your health status. Once employment ceases (or the benefits of employment, such as in a divorce), federal or state law steps in. If your employer is large enough (at least 20 employees), it will usually be covered by federal law.[5] If your employer is not large enough

---

4 A recent U.S. Supreme Court ruling also allows employers to change retiree health benefits, so there is no guarantee that those benefits will be available throughout retirement despite what your employer may be telling you now.

5 The federal law is called the Employees Retirement Income Security Act, or "ERISA."

6 If your employer is not large enough to be covered by ERISA, you may live in a state that provides similar rights for employees of smaller firms, through what is

to be covered by federal law, then your state law will define what—if any—options you will have available to you. [6]

If your employer is covered by federal law, you must make a determination when you leave work whether to accept your "COBRA" coverage.[7] Federal law sets the premium, which will be significantly higher than the premium you may have paid while employed. Under COBRA, the employee is responsible for the *entire* premium plus a 2% administrative charge. After your COBRA rights expire, you have a limited time under the 1996 law, Health Insurance Portability and Accountability Act (HIPAA) to obtain a "guaranteed issue" policy.[8] However, even if HIPAA benefits are offered, there is no guarantee that the benefits will

---

called a "mini-COBRA" law. Some states offer other approaches, and these are often termed "portability" rules.

7 You will be entitled to a limited duration continuation of your employer-sponsored group health benefits under a provision called "COBRA" (Consolidated Omnibus Budget Reconciliation Act). The essential provisions of COBRA are:
▶ If you die or divorce, your spouse can get 36 months of COBRA.
▶ Dependent children who become too old to qualify under the parent's policy can get 36 months of COBRA.
▶ If you apply for Social Security Disability, you can get 29 months of COBRA.
▶ If you become eligible for Medicare, but your spouse is too young to do so, the spouse can get 36 months of COBRA.
▶ You reduce your hours from full-time to part-time and the employer benefits would not otherwise be available in that status, you can get 18 months of COBRA.

8 Be careful, though. HIPAA created a general public impression that anybody who loses or leaves a job has a guaranteed right to get another policy. Keeping coverage under HIPAA is a two-step process; in order to be eligible for a HIPAA-guaranteed issue conversion policy, an employee must first take advantage of COBRA benefits. If COBRA is refused for any reason, then the HIPAA guarantee simply does not apply.

9 The federal HIPAA remedy for this problem can therefore be illusory. Some HIPAA plans are good. However, many are not, and you should check exactly what your HIPAA plan would be before you decide to accept your COBRA. Even if an individual qualifies for a HIPAA conversion plan, the coverage need not resemble what was offered in the employer's group plan, and no affordability limits are placed on premiums for that coverage. Thus, the only individuals who are likely to accept such coverage are those who have essentially no other options, and HIPAA policies are priced accordingly — premiums for such plans can and often do skyrocket when an individual makes claims. Because real protection under the HIPAA federal continuation requirement is essentially illusory, individuals who

---

be equivalent, and there is no limit on premium increases beyond what your state may regulate.[9]

In evaluating your options, check to make sure you know what premium you would have to pay for COBRA benefits. If you choose to bypass your COBRA, then you should make sure that any coverage you obtain in lieu of COBRA would *itself* be continuous.[10] Check renewability and cancellation provisions in individual policies; for group policies, make sure that you know the basis for your own eligibility, and that it is either something you control or which you have satisfactory assurance will continue *throughout your life.*[11] Be aware, however, that COBRA is only for *limited duration.* You should *know before you sign up for COBRA* what your plan for continuation is once the COBRA is over. If you choose to rely upon the HIPAA plan, you should make sure you understand the exact terms of the plan, including any limitations in the benefits, and the extent to which the insurer can raise premiums over the long term.[12] Most states have taken steps to provide some mechanism for individuals to get coverage who cannot obtain insurance in the individual marketplace. In some states, your eligibility

are completely dependent upon employer-sponsored benefits are completely at the mercy of state law, which varies tremendously around the United States. If your HIPAA plan could be a financial disaster, and if accepting your COBRA and, by implication, your HIPAA plan would make you ineligible in your state for other, more reasonable benefits, you should know that before you make a decision about your COBRA.

10 The older you get, the harder it will be to find alternative coverage until you are Medicare eligible. In some states, Medicare supplement insurance—or "Medigap"—is not available at all to individuals who are younger than retirement age. So, if your plan is to get Medicare, make sure you understand whether—or what kind—of supplement would be available to you in your state. If no Medigap is available, then you need to have a plan to meet your expenses that are not covered by Medicare.

11 Most master group insurance contracts have a provision called the "Class of Eligibles" that defines the exact characteristics of the group the insurer has agreed to underwrite. If you are unsure of the basis for your eligibility, you should consult the master contract and look at the language within this provision.

12 You may find that your choice to take the COBRA—and therefore be eligible for HIPAA—limits some of your other choices under state law. This is a serious issue for any person who, for any reason, loses his or her health coverage because of a medical condition.

for a HIPAA plan—no matter how inferior—will disqualify you for any state insurance risk pool.

Thus, a critical set of steps in evaluating your own continuity is to determine—before you have to make the decision about COBRA—what other options for insurance you have.[13] You should check to see what options your state law provides. (For information about your state, go to www.healthinsuranceinfo.net , a website maintained by Georgetown University's Health Policy Institute.)

States offer various approaches to providing coverage for high risk individuals who cannot otherwise obtain coverage in the private marketplace. In some states, there is a designated "insurer of last resort" (such as Blue Cross) that offers specific plans at specific times of the year for open enrollment. The most common approach, taken by more than half of the states, is the offering of a "high risk pool." States understandably discourage reliance on high-risk pools; these pools are far from a panacea and their characteristics vary greatly from state-to-state. Some states cap enrollment; and most do not advertise their programs.[14] Over time, these pools are likely to become more financially squeezed and less reliable. All such pools, of necessity, operate at a loss. Only limited revenues are available to states to operate these pools

13 One insurance product I encourage every American to own that can greatly reduce the effects of employer-sponsored coverage discontinuity is known variously as a "catastrophic excess major medical" or sometimes just as "excess major medical." These products are available in some large groups on a guaranteed issue basis, so they can still be obtained even after a diagnosis of multiple sclerosis, and I encourage every person to have a good one.

14 State risk pools often charge premiums that are high relative to incomes, and typically include sizeable deductibles and copayments, and often restrict annual and lifetime benefits. Even though these pools are designed for people with serious or chronic illnesses, the pools still try to limit enrollment by imposing pre-existing condition exclusions; some are closed to new applicants [including Florida]; and some impose long waiting times [including California and Illinois]. While some states ban HIPAA-eligibles from participating in the pool, other states use the high risk pools to comply with the federal HIPAA, so that the pool becomes the "guaranteed issue" option when your COBRA expires. Some states use their high risk pools as a means of providing Medicare-eligible individuals with a Medicare Supplement, while a few ban enrollment of Medicare eligibles. Because the rules and suitability of the state insurance pools vary tremendously, you should make sure you understand exactly how your own state's pool works.

because self-insured employers are exempt from paying into them. Several proposals before Congress would extend the same exemption to small employers. A good long-term strategy, therefore, should not rely exclusively upon a state high-risk pool as a source for health coverage, if at all possible.

As an alternative to a high-risk pool, some states have made it mandatory for insurance companies to issue coverage to small businesses (sometimes as small as one employee), and have restricted the extent to which premium rates can vary based on health status or age. Thus, another strategy for obtaining insurance, depending upon your state's guarantee issue law, would be to start your own small business.

Non-employment based health insurance

Individuals with MS whose health insurance is not employment-based, who have already retired, or who are attempting to obtain private health insurance for the first time, will need to consider using other products and techniques to protect themselves from the financial risks that accompany medical illness. For our purposes, it is helpful to break down the risks attributable to health-care costs for someone diagnosed with MS into five distinct categories: (1) major medical expenses not due to MS, (2) hospitalization expenses not due to MS, (3) major medical expenses due to MS, (4) hospitalization expenses due to MS, and (5) long-term services expenses.

Many people who have MS find themselves looking for one ideal insurance package to take care of all five of their health-care risks, only to discover that they cannot obtain it after they are diagnosed. That is because MS is considered by the insurance industry to be a serious illness that carries a high risk of associated costs. Therefore, many insurance companies have historically refused to offer coverage to people with MS or have offered it only at a prohibitive cost. Nevertheless, there is no need to subject a person's entire range of healthcare needs to the lowest common denominator of coverage that can be obtained only for a pre-existing, high-risk health condition.

Thus, major medical coverage for conditions other than MS is often the most overlooked component. Just because a member of a family has MS (and therefore may not be able to obtain optimal health coverage for the multiple sclerosis) does not require that all other health needs should be subjected to the common denominator of coverage available for MS. The best way to deal with other health needs is to take a "waiver" or exclusion for MS.[15] In that way, it may be possible to obtain good, thorough, long-term coverage for the person with MS (*without* the MS component) and other members of the family. This strategy requires payment for more than one health policy by the family, but the improvement in coverage should make the investment very worthwhile.

Thus, it often makes more sense to *segregate* your health coverage needs, and seek one good, portable, non–employment-based major medical (and hospitalization) policy for all health risks *except* MS (these are often called policies with "waiver" or "exclusion" provisions). Then, the only risks left to insure would include the risks attributable to MS, and these should be separately insured.

Obtaining major medical coverage for MS is the most difficult challenge for people without employer-sponsored insurance coverage. Nevertheless, a number of strategies are available for persons who cannot obtain insurance through traditional individual sources. If your multiple sclerosis can be considered "benign," then your local insurance agent may be able to find coverage by consulting the book published by National Underwriters entitled "Who Writes What." If not, then you should consult your state options as noted above.

One type of insurance product that can still be obtained (regardless of pre-existing condition) to help cover the excluded MS includes large group "catastrophic" or "excess" major medical. This product will often, after a high deductible has been met (usually approximately $25,000 or $50,000) provide coverage in full for a given condition. Many people are put off by the high deductible; but that is a mistake. These deductibles are not ordinarily measured by the amount that the beneficiary of the policy pays out of pocket; instead they can often be measured by the amounts that *any other insurer* has paid toward a given condition

15 Some states may not make this option available because of underwriting limitations imposed by law.

(including, for example, Medicare, VA, worker's compensation, or private insurance). For example, a $25,000 revolving 36-month deductible simply requires that $25,000 be paid toward a given health condition within a 36-month period by *any accepted payor (including another insurance company)*. If your MS has cost an accumulation of the policy deductible in expenses to all of your payers, you might qualify under the catastrophic plan. In that case, your condition could be declared catastrophic and would be covered (usually at 100% coverage) by the catastrophic plan.

These plans also tend to be quite inexpensive, so it is not difficult to carry them in addition to a regular major medical plan. For example, it is not uncommon to see good major medical coverage with a catastrophic deductible of $25,000 with about $1 million of maximum coverage for an annual premium of less than $200. The "catch" is that usually they are only offered by very large groups, and they often have a waiting period for pre-existing conditions (typically a year or two). Thus, counting backward under such a plan, a person who has MS would have to take out the policy, wait one or two years, and then wait the period while they are accumulating deductible expenses. During this waiting period, other coverage would need to be used for MS-related healthcare costs.

However, if such a plan can be located and locked-in early in the course of the disease, it can often be the "ticket" that gives the person with MS the freedom to avoid catastrophic health insurance–related financial problems as the disease progresses. When combined with any other form of health insurance (including employer-sponsored group major medical), such a plan can reduce the overall exposure to health risks to a fixed amount even in the absence of continuation coverage.

These plans can typically be obtained through large associations or groups. You should check with professional or trade associations, your church, and other types of groups that you are eligible to join to see if such coverage is available.

If you have obtained a good health insurance policy with a waiver or exclusion for your MS, you should have good coverage for hospitalization for conditions unrelated to the disease.

Additionally, if you have obtained a catastrophic major medical policy, hospitalization expenses for your MS may even be covered after any required waiting period and after the catastrophic deductible has been met.

If this strategy is followed, the real gaps in coverage can be limited to include the following: (1) services or expenses that are not traditionally covered by major medical policies, (2) extraordinary expenses you incur that are not strictly health-related, and (3) expenses you may incur while waiting for coverage under one or more of your health plans. Long-term services can be included among the expenses that are not traditionally covered by major medical policies. These nontraditional expenses can also include, for example, the cost of a wheelchair lift system for a van. Depending on your type of insurance, this category may even include all of the costs of a wheelchair. Extraordinary expenses may include such things as extra transportation expenses due to a disability, more meals delivered because of fatigue, or similar expenses. In essence, the "gap" in coverage can simply be thought of as the not-otherwise-covered net additional expenses you incur *precisely because of your MS.*

There is no question that the need for available cash increases as MS progresses. However, contrary to popular opinion, if you find yourself hospitalized fairly frequently for reasons related to MS, you may have a golden opportunity to raise some of that needed cash precisely because you are sick and hospitalized.

One insurance product that is often readily available *even to persons with pre-existing conditions* is called hospital indemnity insurance. This insurance is usually sold to large group associations. It pays fixed amounts or "indemnities" for each day you are hospitalized. These policies have several characteristics that make them attractive under the right conditions:

▶ First, they need not be purchased *before* they become useful. If you are not hospitalized very much, you would be wise merely to begin a file folder with all the information you obtain about any such policies for which you may be eligible. At the appropriate time (discussed next), you can sign up for the various policies.

▶ Second, they tend not to exclude pre-existing conditions. Many of these policies simply have a waiting period for pre-existing conditions.

▶ Third, most of these policies are guaranteed renewable and are issued to large groups. Thus, if you file multiple claims, your future coverage or premiums should not be affected.

▶ Fourth, these policies almost never have limitations or coordination-of-benefits provisions. Thus, they are "stackable." In other words, if it makes financial sense to have one policy, it may make just as much sense to have many such policies. And these policies will usually pay all benefits directly to you, regardless of any other health coverage you may have.

Because these policies will usually pay from approximately $50 per day to approximately $300 per day (some even double the coverage for stays in the intensive care unit), it is not difficult to establish eligibility for thousands of tax-free dollars (assuming that you paid the premiums) every time you are hospitalized. The real trick is to determine *when* to acquire the policies, and *how many* of them you should purchase.

To do this, you need to determine the "index" of the various policies you could obtain. Each policy is usually offered for a fixed annual premium amount. By reading the policy, you can determine how many days of hospitalization it would take to recover your annual premium. For example, if your annual premium is $150, and a proposed policy pays $50 per day beginning on the second day, you would need to be hospitalized for four days to collect your annual premium back in claims benefits. Your "index" for such a policy would be four. For another example, if your policy costs $200 annually, and your policy would pay $125 per day beginning on the third day, you would have to be hospitalized for four days to collect your annual premium back in claims benefits. You should rate each policy similarly, and determine the payment index for each policy.

Next, you need to compare the index scores for each policy to your hospitalization history. When your average annual hospitalization rate exceeds the index on each policy, you should apply for that policy (assuming that it will eventually cover your MS). You should purchase no more policies than you can afford even when you are not hospitalized. Of course, if your average annual hospitalization rate is quite high, and you find yourself receiving large sums, this can be a virtually limitless strategy. Only your imagination in determining what groups you can join to obtain this coverage will limit the amount of cash you can generate when you are ill. Additionally, if the biggest obstacle to your ability to work is hospitalization, this insurance can even serve as a crude substitute for disability insurance.

Unless you find that you are hospitalized often, you need to carry only one of these policies to help pay for the deductibles and co-payments you may have if you are hospitalized. Keep information on the others in a file so that if your amount of hospitalization begins to justify the premiums, you can sign up for multiple policies of this nature at that time.

Estate Planning

A COHESIVE ESTATE plan accomplishes the following things: (1) designates who will get your property when you die; (2) sets up procedures and devices to make sure your property passes to others free from probate, or that your estate owes the least amount possible in probate fees; (3) sets up ways to pass your property to others while reducing or avoiding taxes; and (4) sets up management for property you want to go to others who might need outside help in managing it, including a disabled family member.

Generally, the method you choose to dispose of assets will involve a will, a trust, or both a will and a trust. In using estate planning tools to protect your loved ones, it is advisable to consult an experienced attorney because the law is complex and a mistake might have unfortunate consequences for their future. A common problem overlooked in estate plans is the effect inheritances or gifts can have on eligibility for public benefits. For example, parents who are trying to provide for a disabled child need to be careful not to jeopardize the child's eligibility for public benefits by leaving assets directly in that child's name. In certain circumstances, it may be preferable to limit or eliminate the transfer of assets, so that the child beneficiary is not put in the position of missing out on valuable social services.

Quite often, a will serves as the cornerstone of a financial estate plan. This is a binding legal document that will determine how your estate is distributed after you die.[16] In addition to distributing property, wills can be used to handle certain personal affairs, such as planning funerals and/or making sure that your loved ones are cared for properly if they are legally incompetent or are likely to become incompetent. Parents and guardians can use the will to name their successors. Such designations, depending on the jurisdiction, may be legally binding or of invaluable assistance to a court in guardianship proceedings, should these become necessary. These designees are known as either successor or testamentary guardians.

A trust is a binding legal arrangement in which a person transfers assets to another person, known as a trustee, who manages it for the named beneficiaries. This arrangement may be made as part of a will, in which case it is called a testamentary trust, or it may become effective during your lifetime, in which case it is called a living trust. Additionally, a living trust may be changeable during your lifetime (revocable) or it may be fixed (irrevocable). A trust can be used to select a trustee who will look out for the financial and personal interests of your loved ones without the need for a guardian, and it may result in substantial tax savings. Disadvantages of a trust can include complexity, cost, and the possibility that changing circumstances will leave the trustee without the most appropriate options.

Although trusts may come in many forms, relevant types include:

16 The rules for making a proper will are contained in the laws of each state. If persons die without a will, their property passes by something called "intestate succession," which is a formula determined by state law.

- ▶ Contingent testamentary trust—The proceeds of an estate go first to the surviving spouse but at that spouse's death are placed in trust for a child.
- ▶ Living trust—A pour-over provision that allows property to be added to the trust for the beneficiary once you die.
- ▶ Discretionary trust—Carefully defines the amount and kind of discretion that the trustee will have in distributing or withholding benefits; (in many states, a particular type of discretionary trust called a special needs or supplemental need trust can be established to meet the needs of a disabled child over and above the needs met through government benefits. This trust is designed in such a way that it will add to government benefits without jeopardizing the beneficiary's eligibility for those benefits).
- ▶ Sprinkling trust—Allows you to instruct the trustee to distribute the benefits unequally according to the unique needs of the beneficiaries.
- ▶ Life insurance trust—Helps ensure that the benefits of a life insurance policy will be managed properly.

It is in your best interests to consult an estate planning attorney in order to make sure that you are pursuing the most suitable option(s), given your financial and social circumstances, so that you loved ones will be protected both financially and socially once you pass away.

Conclusion

A THOROUGH LIFE plan is a necessary strategy for protecting your family and avoiding many of the pitfalls that could rob you of your security or freedom. This chapter provides an overview of the process as well as some options for you and your family to consider. Fortunately, there are now available a number of resources to guide you through the process. Please see the Recommended Resources and Additional Readings provided at the end of this book and consult a qualified professional in your area.

ADDITIONAL READINGS

Bove A. *The Medicaid Planning Handbook: A Guide to Protecting Your Family's Assets from Catastrophic Nursing Home Costs* (2nd ed.) Boston: Little, Brown (TimeWarner), 1996.

Epstein R. *Maximizing Your Health Insurance Benefits: A Consumer's Guide to New and Traditional Plans.* Westport, CT: Praeger (Greenwood Publishing Group), 1997.

Exceptional Parent Magazine. *The EP [Exceptional Parent] Resource Guide 2004.* Available online at http://www.eparent.com/resourceguide2004/index.htm.

Landay D. *Be Prepared: The Complete Financial, Legal, and Practical Guide for Living with a Life-Challenging Condition.* Hampshire, England: St. Martins Press (Palgrave MacMillan), 2000.

Northrop D, Cooper S. *Health Insurance Resources: Options for People with a Chronic Disease or Disability.* New York: Demos Medical Publishing, 2003.

Russell LM, Grant AE. *The Life Planning Workbook: A Hands-On Guide to Help Parents Provide for the Future Security and Happiness of Their Child with Disability After Their Death.* American Publishing Company, 1995.

Scholen K. *Reverse Mortgages for Beginners: A Consumer Guide to Every Homeowner's Retirement Nest Egg.* NCHE Press, 1998.

Stevens B. *The ABC's of Special Needs Planning Made Easy.* Stevens Group Lic., 2002.

RECOMMENDED RESOURCE [INTERNET]

Laura's Links: http://www.lauraslinks.com/Links1.htm [Laura Cooper's website of links designed to assist individuals with their insurance planning]

13

Supportive Resources for Families

Nancy Holland, RN, EdD
Kimberly Koch, MPA
Deborah Hertz, MPH

Over the past several years, many kinds of MS resources have emerged to help families cope with the challenges of multiple sclerosis [see Appendices A and B for additional readings and resources]. This chapter will familiarize you with the types of resources that are available and encourage you to think of them as valuable tools to use in your coping efforts. Whether these resources take the form of reading materials, support groups, counseling, or educational programs, their value lies in providing families with the information and support they need to adapt more comfortably to the changes that MS brings into their lives. Because no family is likely to use all of the available resources, this discussion presents you with a menu of available options that your family can use now and in the future.

It is important to remember that even within the same family, people tend to vary in their styles of learning and coping. No two people are exactly alike in their responses to stress, change, or loss. In addition, each person's needs may shift over time as a result of personal growth and development, a change in circumstances, or even education. These differences must be taken into account when the family seeks assistance in dealing with the complexities of MS. Sometimes the family may seek information and support together, via shared reading, family workshops, or family counseling. At other times, however, individual family members may opt for different courses of action that provide them with the most comfortable means of gathering information and getting emotional support. Thus, one person might decide to attend a National Multiple Sclerosis Society educational program, another might choose to read a few brief pamphlets, and a third might select the option of one-on-one interaction with a health professional or a person in a similar MS family situation. There is no "correct" way to learn about MS or to cope with its impact on family life. Each family, and each individual within the family, needs to consider the available resources in the way that feels most useful to them.

Psychoeducational Resources

THE TERM *psychoeducational* refers to the important interaction between learning and coping functions. Ideally, families should be gathering accurate, up-to-date information about MS at the same time that they are dealing with their emotional reactions to its presence in the household. Experience has repeatedly demonstrated the effectiveness of knowledge and understanding as coping tools. Obtaining information about MS and the various ways in which it can impact family life enables individuals and families to feel more in control and more prepared to deal with this chronic, unpredictable disease.

Psychoeducational activities include educational programs (sponsored by the National MS Society and other organizations), participation in workshops of different kinds, support groups, counseling, and less formal interactions with an MS expert— either a professional or a peer (a person who has MS or a family member with training to provide appropriate information about personal experiences with MS). Again, the combined function of any of these activities is to provide useful information in a supportive style and setting.

Educational Programs and Materials

THE NATIONAL MS Society offers a wide variety of programs and reading materials for individuals with MS and their families (Call 1-800-FIGHT-MS; 1-800-344-4867 to reach the chapter in your area). From the time of diagnosis onward, these programs and materials are designed to meet the needs of persons with MS, their spouses or partners, and their children.

- ► Information about MS, treatment strategies, recent research developments, and education and support programs can be found on the National MS Society's website http://www.nationalmssociety.org. Archived Web broadcasts and conferences are available in the Living with MS section of the website. Web spotlights, highlighting information on the website on a wide range of topics, can be accessed at http://www.nationalmssociety.org/Spotlight.asp.
- ► Pamphlets and booklets on virtually every aspect of living with MS (including some specifically designed for people who are newly diagnosed and for children who have a parent with MS) can be obtained by calling 1-800-FIGHT-MS or downloaded from the library section of the website at http://www.nationalmssociety.org/Library.asp.
- ► *Keep S'myelin* is a free newsletter for children, ages 6-12, who have a parent with MS. Each issue contains stories related to a specific MS issue, games and activities, and a parents' pull-out section with information and resources to help parents talk with their children about MS. To subscribe or receive copies of back issues, call 1-800-FIGHT-MS (1-800-344-4867). Interactive versions of *Keep S'myelin* are available in the library section of the website at http://www.nationalmssociety.org/Library.asp.
- ► The *Journey Club*, a chapter-sponsored education program for parents with MS and their children (ages 5-12), is designed to help parents and children discuss issues related to the family's journey with MS, including symptoms, emotional reactions, changes in family life, and support systems. The program provides parents and children with opportunities

to voice their concerns, dispel misunderstandings and myths about MS, and learn about the disease together. It also helps parents develop strategies for meeting the challenges of parenting with MS.

▶ *Young Persons with MS—A Network for Families with a Child or Teen with MS* provides the opportunity for families with a child with MS to learn more about pediatric MS and connect with other families living with the disease. Although children make up less than 1% of the MS population, the need for these children and their families to connect with others in the same circumstances can be quite intense. Services of the network include teleconferences, a handbook for parents, and short-term counseling. To learn more about the Network, call 1-866 KIDS W MS (1-866-543-7967) or e-mail childhoodms@nmss.org.

▶ *Mighty Special Kids—An Activity Book for Children with MS.* This activity book is for children 5-12 who have MS. It includes educational games, activities, and age appropriate articles to help children better understand their diagnosis. Parents can request the book by calling 1-866-KIDS or by emailing childhoodms@nmss.org.

▶ Chapter-sponsored children's camps provide youngsters who have a parent with MS the opportunity to meet in a fun and relaxing atmosphere. The children learn about MS while enjoying a short vacation from it.

▶ Conferences sponsored by chapters of the National MS Society offer opportunities for people with MS and their family members to hear presentations on various topics, participate in workshops, and meet others who are living and coping with MS.

▶ Chapter-sponsored *Family Days* are programs specially designed to meet the psychoeducational needs of parents and children.

▶ The cartoon for children entitled *Timmy's Journey to Understanding MS* is available from chapters for home viewing.

▶ Each chapter of the National MS Society has a lending library that provides books, audiotapes, and videotapes that are of interest to families living with MS. (Individual chapters can be reached by calling the Society's national toll-free number.)

In addition to educational programs sponsored by the National MS Society, there may be others available through local MS care centers. Call 1-800-FIGHT-MS to find out if there is a center in your area that is affiliated with the National MS Society and/or the Consortium of MS Centers (CMSCs—an organization of centers throughout the United States and Canada that disseminates information to clinicians and advances the standard of care in MS). The CMSC can also be contacted directly by calling the headquarters located at the Gimbel MS Center in Teaneck, New Jersey (201-837-0727).

Apart from the materials available from the National MS Society, there are several up-to-date books on MS, including more general reference books and those that target specific aspects of MS management (see Appendix A for Additional Readings). Whether or not reading is the primary learning choice of individual family members, it is useful to have one or more reference texts on hand for everyone to use. This provides immediate answers to questions, as well as a starting point for discussion of various topics. Although there are usually several ways to answer any given question, the family will find it helpful to have one main reference point with which to compare contrasting opinions from other sources. One comprehensive reference—*Multiple Sclerosis: The Questions You Have—The Answers You Need* (3rd ed.), compiled by the editor of this book, offers information about a wide range of topics in a question-and-answer format, an extensive glossary, listings of recommended readings and resources, and a section that contains medication information sheets.

Another reference that focuses on personal control and independence is *Multiple Sclerosis: A Self-Care Guide to Wellness* (2nd ed.), also available from Demos Medical Publishing. The authors of this book have used the wellness model to provide readers with a broad knowledge of MS and its implications for an individual's overall health and well-being. It discusses self-care and general wellness activities that are designed to promote maximal comfort, independence, and productivity.

Self-Help Groups

SELF-HELP (SUPPORT) groups exist in almost every section of the country, with over 1,800 groups affiliated with the National MS Society. Group leaders (either professionals or peers) have participated in the Society's training programs to enhance their skills in active listening, group dynamics, problem-solving guidance, crisis intervention, and other important areas. Groups vary enormously in the profile of members (e.g., newly diagnosed, more severely disabled, caregivers) and target a variety of concerns including coping and adaptation, employment issues, parenting, and so forth. Self-help groups may have emotional support as their primary focus, or may combine this with education, advocacy, and social activities. The frequency of meetings ranges from weekly to monthly. Meetings may be carried out by telephone or in the more common, in-person format. To find a Society-sponsored group in your area, call 1-800-FIGHT-MS.

Counseling

COUNSELING BY HEALTHCARE professionals (e.g., psychologists, social workers, family therapists, or nurses) is designed to support people's efforts to live and cope with the stress and turmoil caused by MS. Unfortunately, many people still perceive counseling as an activity for the emotionally weak or unstable, and therefore shy away from this helpful resource. In the same way that one would not build a house without power tools, one should not try to learn how to live with MS without tools such as information, guidance, and support. Counseling is an avenue for obtaining all of these. Within the supportive setting of counseling, individuals, couples, and whole families can receive answers to their questions, gain insight into their feelings and reactions, talk more openly about their reactions to the intrusion of MS in their lives, learn more effective coping strategies and communication skills, and problem-solve in areas of their lives that are causing them concern.

MS typically involves a variety of symptoms that ebb and flow over the course of the illness. Whether someone remains relatively stable or gradually becomes more disabled, these symptoms can have an impact on self-esteem and emotional well-being, family life, employment, and overall quality of life. When individuals or families feel overwhelmed by uncomfortable feelings or unavoidable changes in their lives, it is often difficult to identify available options and make satisfying choices. Counseling can facilitate this process—whether it be a single consultation or several sessions over the course of the illness. During any period of major change or stress, one or another form of counseling can support the efforts of an individual or the whole family to regain a sense of emotional balance and control.

Different people will opt to make use of counseling in different ways—perhaps for help at the time of diagnosis, for sorting out family-related decisions or a job change, for occasional support in the event of a crisis, or on a more long-term basis. Counseling can take a variety of forms, but the overall goal is always to support people's efforts to enhance their quality of life.

▶ Individual counseling allows the person with MS or a family member to become more informed about MS, explore feelings and concerns, identify options, enhance current coping strategies and/or develop new ones, and receive emotional support. In this type of counseling, people develop an understanding of the grieving process that necessarily accompanies the life changes brought about by MS. For some individuals, the opportunity to explore feelings in a one-on-one situation with a therapist lays the groundwork for participation in support groups or family therapy.

▶ Group counseling provides a forum for people to share information and problem-solving strategies, provide mutual support, and enjoy the experience of being with others who are "in the same boat." Group counseling is available not only for individuals with MS, but also for well-spouses, couples, children who have a parent with MS, or any other set of individuals with a shared agenda (e.g., working parents, people with cognitive impairment). Within the group setting, people find they can talk and laugh about problems that would be too personal to talk about in other situations.

They can express feelings of anger, resentment, or fear that they might hesitate to share with family members or friends. Most importantly, perhaps, the group setting encourages the development of relationships that continue to provide a valuable social support network long after the group sessions are completed. Group counseling by telephone is also available in some areas for people with severe disabilites or who are limited by geography or fatigue from attending a group session in person.

▶ Family counseling helps families recognize the impact of MS on family life, communicate more comfortably with one another about their reactions to the illness, identify and understand the varying coping styles of individual family members, and problem-solve more effectively. A major goal of family counseling is to help the family learn how to adapt to the presence of MS in the household without allowing the disease to drain more of the family's emotional resources than it needs.

Community Resources

IN ADDITION TO the National MS Society, there are a variety of community resources available to meet the needs of families living with MS. To find out about agencies in your area that serve children and families, contact your local chapter of United Way. Examples of national organizations include:

▶ **Multiple Sclerosis Society of Canada** (175 Bloor Street East, Suite 700, North Tower, Toronto, Ontario M4W 3R8; Tel: 1-416-922-6065 or 1-800-268-7582; Website: www.mssociety.ca). The services and programs of the regional divisions and chapters include: information and referral; educational conferences and workshops; support programs; advocacy; assistance programs.

▶ **National Family Caregivers Association** (10400 Connecticut Avenue #500, Kensington, MD 20895; Tel: 1-800-896-3650; Website: www.thefamilycaregiver.org). NFCA is dedicated to improving quality of life for America's 18,000,000 caregivers. It publishes a quarterly newsletter and has a resource guide, information clearing house, and a toll-free hotline.

► **Through the Looking Glass: National Research and Training Center on Families of Adults with Disabilities** (2198 Sixth Street, Suite 100, Berkeley, CA 94710-2204; Tel: 1-510- 848-1112 or 1-800-644-2666; Website: http://lookingglass.org). The Center offers a free quarterly newsletter on parenting with a disability.

► **United Spinal Association (formerly the Eastern Paralyzed Veterans Association)** (75-20 Astoria Boulevard, Jackson Heights, NY 11370; Tel: 1-718-803-3782 or 1-800-807-0192; Website: www.unitedspinal.org. While maintaining its commitment to veterans, USA assists all people with spinal cord injury or disease by ensuring quality health care, promoting research, and advocating for civil rights and independence. They publish a quarterly newsletter, *MS Quarterly Report*, and have programs to assist members improve home accessibility.

► **Well Spouse Association** (P.O. Box 801, New York, NY 10023; Tel: 1-212-685-8815 or 1-800-838-0879; Website: www.wellspouse.org). This membership organization offers an emotional support network for the significant others of persons with a chronic illness. The services offered by the Foundation include advocacy for home health and long-term care, peer support, and a newsletter.

The Internet offers the opportunity for individuals with MS or their family members to share information, support, and problem-solving ideas with others who are in a similar situation. This has proved to be an invaluable resource, particularly for people with severe disabilities or who have limited access to MS facilities in their area.

Summary

BECOMING MORE INFORMED about MS enables people to understand the potential impact of the disease on daily life, family relationships, and everyone's emotional well-being. Taking advantage of the available psychoeducational resources is one important way for people who have the disease and their family members to reduce anxiety, gain a greater sense of control, and feel more comfortable in their everyday lives. In addition, the knowledge gained about the disease and its management helps people cope more effectively now and in the future.

Learning about the disease and its potential impact on family life will enable you to recognize stresses and problems as they arise. The resources described in this chapter exist to help you cope with today, anticipate tomorrow's difficulties, and develop strategies to avert family crises. There is no need to wait for a crisis to develop before getting help. Needing assistance is not unique to families living with MS—we all need support at different times in our lives. Check out the resources in this chapter and discuss your concerns with your physician or other healthcare provider (e.g., a nurse, social worker, or psychologist). Tracking down the appropriate support person or service may sometimes be frustrating, but be persistent. The important first step is the decision to look for the help you need.

APPENDIX A

Additional Readings

Books from Demos Medical Publishing

Bowling A. *Alternative Medicine and Multiple Sclerosis*, 2001.

Coyle PK, Halper J. *Meeting the Challenges of Progressive Multiple Sclerosis*, 2001.

Davis A. *My Story: A Photographic Essay on Life with Multiple Sclerosis*, 2004.

Giffels JJ. *Clinical Trials: What You Should Know Before Volunteering to Be a Research Subject*, 1996.

Holland N, Halper J, (eds.) *Multiple Sclerosis: A Self-Care Guide to Wellness* (2nd ed.), 2005.

Holland N, Murray TJ, Reingold SC. *Multiple Sclerosis: A Guide for the Newly Diagnosed* (2nd ed.), 2001. [Spanish translation: Esclerosis Multiple: Guia Practica Para el Recien Diagnosticado, 2002].

Kalb R, (ed.) *Multiple Sclerosis: The Questions You Have; The Answers You Need* (3rd ed.), 2004.

Kraft GH, Catanzaro M. *Living with Multiple Sclerosis: A Wellness Approach* (2nd ed.), 2000.

Kramer D. *Life on Cripple Creek: Essays on Living with Multiple Sclerosis*, 2003.

Murray J. *Multiple Sclerosis: The History of a Disease*, 2004.

Nichols J. *Women Living with Multiple Sclerosis*, 1999.

Nichols J. *Living Beyond Multiple Sclerosis: A Women's Guide*, 2000

Northrop D, Cooper S. *Insurance Resources: Options for People with a Chronic Illness or Disability*, 2003.

Perkins L, Perkins S. *Multiple Sclerosis: Your Legal Rights* (2nd ed.), 1999.

Rumrill PD, Jr. (ed.) *Employment Issues and Multiple Sclerosis*, 1996.

Schapiro RT. *Symptom Management in Multiple Sclerosis* (4th ed.), 2003.

Schwarz SP. *300 Tips for Making Life with Multiple Sclerosis Easier*, 1999.

Other Books

Alliance for Technology Access. *Computer and Web Resources for People with Disabilities: A Guide to Exploring Today's Assistive Technology.* Hunter House, Inc., 2001. [ordering@hunterhouse.com].

Baldacci S. *A Sundog Moment.* Warner Faith, 2004.

Barrett M. *Sexuality and Multiple Sclerosis.* 3rd ed. Toronto: Multiple Sclerosis Society of Canada, 1991.

Barrett S, Jarvis WT, (eds.) *The Health Robbers: A Close Look at Quackery in America.* Buffalo: Prometheus Books, 1993.

Blackstone M. *First Year—Multiple Sclerosis: An Essential Guide for the Newly Diagnosed.* New York: Marlowe and Co., 2002. [www.marlowepub.com].

Carroll DL, Dorman JD. *Living Well with MS: A Guide for Patient, Caregiver, and Family.* New York: HarperCollins, 1993.

Cassileth BR. *The Alternative Medicine Handbook.* New York: W.W. Norton & Co., 1998.

Chapman B. *Coping with Vision Loss: Maximizing What You Can See and Do.* Alameda, CA: Hunter House, 2001. [ordering@hunterhouse.com].

Cohen MD. *Dirty Details.* Philadelphia: Temple University Press, 1996.

Cohen, RM. *Blindsided: Lifting a Life above Illness: A Reluctant Memoir.* New York: HarperCollins, 2004.

Cristall B. *Coping When a Parent has Multiple Sclerosis.* New York: Rosen Publishing, 1992. [written for teens].

Dohrmann V. *Treating Memory Impairments: A Memory Book and Other Strategies.* Tucson, AZ: Communication Skill Builders, 1994.

Donoghue PJ, Siegel ME. *Sick and Tired of Feeling Sick and Tired: Living with Invisible Chronic Illness.* New York: WW Norton, 1992.

Fennell P. *The Chronic Illness Workbook.* New Harbinger Publications, Inc., 2001 [available at www.amazon.com].

Garee B, (ed.) *Parenting: Tips from Parents (Who Happen to Have a Disability) on Raising Children.* Bloomington, IL: Accent Press, 1989.

Harrington, C. *Barrier-Free Travel: A Nuts and Bolts Guide for Wheelers and Slow Walkers.* C & C Creative Concepts, 2001. [EmergingHorizons.com/book].

Hecker H. *Travel for the Disabled: A Handbook of Travel Resources and 500 Worldwide Access Guides.* Vancouver, WA: Twin Peaks Press, 1995.

Hill B. *Multiple Sclerosis Q & A: Reassuring Answers to Frequently Asked Questions.* Avery Penguin Putnam, 2003.

Iezzoni LI. *When Walking Fails.* Berkeley: University of California Press, 2003.

James JL. *One Particular Harbor: The Outrageous True Adventures of One Woman with Multiple Sclerosis Living in the Alaskan Wilderness.* Chicago: Noble Press, 1993.

Kaufman M, Silverberg C, Odette F. *The Ultimate Guide to Sex and Disability.* San Francisco: Cleis Press, 2003.

Kroll K, Klein EL. *Enabling Romance: A Guide to Love, Sex, and Relationships for the Disabled.* Bethesda, MD: Woodbine House, 1995.

Lander D. *Fall Down Laughing.* Putnam Publishing Group, 2000.

MacFarlane EB, Burstein P. *Legwork: An Inspiring Journey through a Chronic Illness.* New York: Charles Scribner's Sons, 1994.

Mackenzie L, (ed.) *The Complete Directory for the Disabled.* Lakeville, CT: Grey House Publishing, Inc., 1991.

Mairs N. *Waist-High in the World: A Life Among the Nondisabled.* Beacon Press, 1998.

Matthews J. *Beat the Nursing Home Trap: A Consumer's Guide to Choosing and Financing Long-Term Care.* 2nd ed. Berkeley, CA: Nolo Press, 1993

Mintz SB. *Love, Honor, and Value: A Family Caregiver Speaks out about the Choices and Challenges of Caregiving.* Capital Books, Inc., 2002.

Neistadt ME, Freda M. *Choices: A Guide to Sex Counseling with Physically Disabled Adults.* Malabar, FL: Robert E. Krieger Publishing Co., 1987.

Pitzele SK. *We Are Not Alone: Learning to Live with Chronic Illness.* New York: Workman Publishing, 1986.

Pitzele SK. *One More Day: Daily Meditations for the Chronically Ill.* Minnesota: Hazelden, 1988.

Price J. *Avoiding Attendants from Hell: A Practical Guide to Funding, Hiring, and Keeping Personal Care Attendants.* Science and Humanities Press, 1998. [www.banis-associates.com].

Resources for Rehabilitation. *Resources for People with Disabilities and Chronic Conditions* (5th ed.) Winchester, MA: Resources for Rehabilitation, 2002.

Resources for Rehabilitation. *A Man's Guide to Coping with Disability* (3rd ed.) Winchester, MA: Resources for Rehabilitation, 2003.

Resources for Rehabilitation. *A Woman's Guide to Coping with Disability* (4th ed.) Winchester, MA: Resources for Rehabilitation, 2003.

Resources for Rehabilitation. *Living with Low Vision: A Resource Guide for People with Sight Loss* (6th ed.) Winchester, MA: Resources for Rehabilitation, 2001.

Resources for Rehabilitation. *Making Wise Medical Decisions: How to Get the Information You Need* (2nd ed.) Winchester, MA: Resources for Rehabilitation, 2001

Resources for Rehabilitation. *Meeting the Needs of Employees with Disabilities* (4th ed.) Winchester, MA: Resources for Rehabilitation, 2004.

Russell LM, Grant AE, Joseph SM, Fee RW. *Planning for the Future: Providing a Meaningful Life for a Child with a Disability After Your Death* (2nd ed.) Evanston, IL: American Publishing, 1995.

Russell M, (ed.) *When the Road Turns: Inspirational Stories By and About People with MS.* Health Communications, Inc., 2001. [http://www.hci-online.com].

Spero D. *The Art of Getting Well: A Five-Step Plan for Maximizing Health When You Have a Chronic Illness.* Alameda, CA: Hunter House, 2002. [ordering@hunterhouse.com].

Sohlberg M, Mateer C. *Introduction to Cognitive Rehabilitation: Theory and Practice.* New York: Guilford Press.

Strong M. *Mainstay: For the Well Spouse of the Chronically Ill.* Bradford Books, 1997.

Tyler VE. *The Honest Herbal* (4th ed.) New York: Haworth Press, 1998.

Winks C, Semans A. *The Good Vibrations Guide to Sex* (3rd ed.) San Francisco: Cleis Press, 2004.

Wright LM, Leahey M. *Families and Chronic illness.* Philadelphia: Spring House, 1987.

Yaffe M, Fenwick E, Rosen RC, Kellett JM. *Sexual Happiness for Women: A Practical Approach.* New York: Henry Holt & Co., 1992.

Yaffe M, Fenwick E, Rosen RC, Kellett JM. *Sexual Happiness for Men: A Practical Approach.* New York: Henry Holt & Co., 1992.

Publications Available from
The National Multiple Sclerosis Society

The National MS Society offers a comprehensive selection of booklets, brochures, magazines, and other materials about multiple sclerosis. To view and download these publications, visit the Library (http://www. nationalmssociety.org/Library.asp) on the Society's website. Or, you can request these materials from your chapter of the Society by calling 1-800-FIGHT-MS (1-800-344-4867).

General Information

Just the Facts 2003-2004
Research Directions in Multiple Sclerosis
Choosing the Right Health-Care Provider
The History of Multiple Sclerosis
Living with MS
Putting the Brakes on MS
What Everyone Should Know About Multiple Sclerosis
What Is Multiple Sclerosis?

Employment Issues

ADA and People with MS
Information for Employers
A Place in the Workforce
Should I Work? Information for Employees
The Win-Win Approach to Reasonable Accommodations: Enhancing Productivity on
       Your Job

For the Newly Diagnosed

Comparing the Disease–Modifying Drugs
Diagnosis: The Basic Facts
Disclosure: The Basic Facts
Genetics: The Basic Facts
Living with MS
Putting the Brakes on MS

Staying Well

Clear Thinking about Alternative Therapies
Dental Health: The Basic Facts
Exercise as Part of Everyday Life
Food for Thought: MS and Nutrition
Managing MS Through Rehabilitation
Multiple Sclerosis and Your Emotions
Preventive Care Recommendations for Adults with MS: The Basic Facts
Stretching for People with MS
Stretching with a Helper for People with MS
Taming Stress in Multiple Sclerosis
Vitamins, Minerals, and Herbs in MS: An Introduction

Managing Specific Issues

Bowel Problems: The Basic Facts
"But You Look So Good!"
Controlling Bladder Problems in Multiple Sclerosis
Controlling Spasticity in MS
Depression and Multiple Sclerosis
Fatigue: What You Should Know
Gait or Walking Problems: The Basic Facts
Hormones: The Basic Facts
MS and Intimacy
MS and the Mind
MS and Pregnancy
Pain: The Basic Facts
Sleep Disorders and MS: The Basic Facts
Solving Cognitive Problems
Speech and Swallowing: The Basic Facts
Tremor: The Basic Facts
Urinary Dysfunction and MS
Vision Problems: The Basic Facts

Managing Major Changes

At Home with MS: Adapting Your Environment
A Guide for Caregivers
Hiring Help at Home: The Basic Facts
Managing Progressive MS
PLAINTALK: A Booklet About MS for Families
So You Have Progressive MS?

For Children and Teenagers

Keep S'myelin—A quarterly newsletter for children ages 6–12 who have
    a parent with MS—available in hard copy or in the Society's
    online library at http://www.nationalmssociety.org/library.asp
When a Parent Has MS: A Teenager's Guide
Teen InsideMS Online—A quarterly online magazine
(*nationalmssociety.org/Teen%20InsideMS.asp*)
Someone You Know Has MS: A Booklet for Families

Materials Available in Spanish

Comparación de los Medicamentos Modificadores de la
    Enfermedad
Controlando los Problemas de la Vejiga en la Esclerosis Múltiple
Debo Trabajar? Información para Empleados
Diagnóstico: Hechos Básicos sobre Esclerosis Múltiple
Ejercicios Prácticos de Estiramiento para las Personas con Esclerosis
    Múltiple
Ejercicios Prácticos de Estiramiento con un Ayudante para las
    Personas con
Esclerosis Múltiple
La Fatigua: Lo Que Usted Debe Saber
Información para Empleadores
Lo Que Todo el Mundo Debe Saber Sobre la Esclerosis Múltiple
"¡Pero si te ves tan bien!"
¿Qué es la Esclerosis Múltiple?
Sobre los Problemas Sexuales Que No Mencionan los Médicos

Other National MS Society Publications:

Inside MS—A 32-page magazine for people living with MS published three times yearly

Knowledge is Power—a series of articles for individuals newly diagnosed with MS

Canadian Multiple Sclerosis Society Publication (1-416-922-6065)

Coping with Fatigue in MS Takes Understanding and Planning—Alexander Burnfield, M.B., M.R.C. Psych.

Eastern Paralyzed Veterans Association Publications (1-800-444-0120)

Single copies of the following publications are available in print, based on supply at the time of order. Many are also available for downloading in HTML format at http://data.unitedspinal.org/Publications/Publications.asp.

- ▶ Access State and Local Government (Title II)—Summarizes the rights of people with disabilities and the responsibilities of state and local governments under the ADA (Title II). Includes a compliance checklist.
- ▶ Accessible Air Travel—A handy guide that explains the Air Carrier Access and provides information about air travel for wheelchair users.
- ▶ Disability Etiquette—Provides pointers on how to relate to people with various disabilities.
- ▶ Taking Action—A step-by-step, self-help guide to becoming a self-advocate and making a difference (also available in Spanish).
- ▶ Understanding the ADA—Details the most important provisions of the ADA as well as the available tax incentives for small businesses that remove barriers for people with disabilities.

General Publications

- ▶ *Access to Travel*—A quarterly magazine published by the Society for the Advancement of Travel for the Handicapped (SATH). A nonprofit organization that works to create a barrier-free environment throughout the travel and tourism industry (347 Fifth Avenue, Suite 610, New York, NY 10016; 212-447-7284).

APPENDIX B

Recommended Resources

THIS LIST OF resources is designed to help you and your family meets the challenges of multiple sclerosis. While no means complete, it can serve as a starting point; each resource that you investigate will lead you to others and they, in turn, will lead you to even more.

Information Sources

Clearinghouse on Disability Information, Communications and Information Services, Office of Special Education and Rehabilitative Services, U.S. Department of Education, (Switzer Building, 330 C Street, S.W., Washington, D.C. 20202; tel: 800-872-5327; Internet: www.ed. gov/about/offices/list/osers/index.html). Created by the Rehabilitation Act of 1973, the Clearinghouse responds to inquiries about federal laws, services, and programs for individuals of all ages with disabilities.

Disability Rights Education and Defense Fund, Inc. (DREDF) (2212 Sixth Street, Berkeley, CA 94710; tel: 510-644-2555; 800-466-4232; Internet: www.dredf.org; e-mail: dredf@dredf.org). DREDF is a national law and policy center dedicated to furthering the civil rights of people with disabilities. The center provides assistance, information, and referrals on disability rights laws; legal representation in cases involving civil rights; and education/training for legislators, policy makers, and law students.

Easter Seals/March of Dimes National Council (90 Eglinton Avenue East, Suite 511, Toronto, Ontario M4P 2Y3, Canada; tel: 416-932-8382; Internet: www.esmodnc.org; e-mail: national.council@esmodnc.org). The Council is a federation of regional and provincial groups serving individuals with disabilities throughout Canada. It operates an information service and publishes a newsletter and a quarterly journal.

Inglis House (2600 Belmont Avenue, Philadelphia, PA 19131; tel: 215-878-5600; Internet: www.inglis.org). A national information exchange network specializing in long-term facilities for mentally alert persons with physical disabilities.

National Health Information Center (P.O. Box 1133, Washington, D.C. 20013; tel: 800-336-4797; Internet: www.health.gov/nhic). The Center maintains a library and a database of health-related organizations. It also provides referrals related to health issues for consumers and professionals.

President's Committee on Employment of People with Disabilities (1331 F Street, N.W., Washington, D.C. 20004-1107; tel: 202-376-6200). The Committee publishes employment-related brochures for individuals with disabilities and their employers, and provides the Job Accommodation Network (tel: 800-526-7234).

Electronic Information Sources

There are many sources of information available free through the Internet on the World Wide Web. If you are an experienced net surfer, switch to your favorite search facility and enter the keywords "MS" or "multiple sclerosis." This will generally give you a listing of dozens of websites that pertain to MS. Keep in mind, however, that the World Wide Web is a free and open medium; while many of the websites have excellent and useful information, others may contain highly unusual and inaccurate information. Following is a list of some recommended MS sites available through the Internet. Each of these will provide links to other sites.

ABLEDATA
Information on Assistive Technology
http://www.abledata.com/

Allsup, Inc.
Assists individuals applying for Social Security Disability benefits
http://www.allsupinc.com/

Apple Computer Disability Resources
http://www.apple.com/education/k12/disability/

Avonex®
http://www.avonex.com/

Betaseron®
http://www.betaseron.com/

CenterWatch Clinical Trials Listing Service(tm)
http://www.centerwatch.com/

CLAMS—Computer Literate Advocates for Multiple Sclerosis
http://www.clams.org/

Consortium of Multiple Sclerosis Centers
http://www.mscare.org/

Copaxone®
http://www.copaxone.com/

Disabled Online
A website dedicated to providing beneficial resources for the disabled
community and their families and friends http://www.disabledon
line.com/

The Heuga Program
A program emphasizing health, physical fitness, and psychological well-
being
www.heuga.org

IBM Accessibility Center
http://www.ibm.com/able/

Infosci
Selected links on MS

http://www.infosci.org/

International Federation of Multiple Sclerosis Societies/The World of
    Multiple Sclerosis
http://www.nmss.org/

International Journal of MS Care
http://www.mscare.com/

Medicare Information
http://www.medicare.com

Microsoft Accessibility Technology for Everyone
http://www.microsoft.com/enable/

MS Crossroads
Personal Website of Aapo Halko, Ph.D., mathematician with MS in
    Finland
http://www.mscrossroads.org

The Multiple Sclerosis Information Gateway
Schering AG, Berlin, Germany
http://www.ms-gateway.com/

Multiple Sclerosis Society of Canada
http://www.mssociety.ca/

Myelin Project
http://www.myelin.org/

National Family Caregivers Association
http://www.thefamilycaregiver.org/

National Institute of Neurological Disorders and Stroke
http://www.ninds.nih.gov/

National Library of Medicine
http://www.nlm.nih.gov/

National Multiple Sclerosis Society
http://www.nationalmssociety.org/

National Organization for Rare Disorders
http://www.rarediseases.org/

NARIC—The National Rehabilitation Information Center
http://www.naric.com/

Novantrone®
http://www.novantrone.com

Rebif®
http://www.rebif.com

Resource Materials

Assistive Technology Sourcebook. (Written by A. Enders and M. Hall, published by Resna Press, Washington, D.C. 1990).

The Complete Directory for People with Chronic Illness, 1998–1999 (published by Grey House Publishing, Inc., 185 Millerton Road, P.O. Box 860, Millerton, NY 12546; tel: 800-562-2139; fax: 860-435-3004; Internet: www.greyhouse.com; e-mail: books@greyhouse.com).

The Complete Directory for People with Disabilities, 1999–2000 (published by Grey House Publishing, Inc., 185 Millerton Road, P.O. Box 860, Millerton, NY 12546; tel: 800-562-2139; fax: 860-435-3004; Internet: www.greyhouse.com; e-mail: books@greyhouse.com).

Complete Drug Reference. (Compiled by United States Pharmacopoeia, published by Consumer Report Books, A division of Consumers Union, Yonkers, NY.) This comprehensive, readable, and easy-to-use drug reference includes almost every prescription and non-prescription medication available in the United States and Canada. A new edition is published yearly.

Dressing Tips and Clothing Resources for Making Life Easier. (Written by Shelly Peterman Schwarz, c/o Real Living with MS, 1111 Bethlehem Pike, P.O. Box 908, Springhouse, PA 19477).

Exceptional Parent: Parenting Your Child or Young Adult with a Disability. A monthly magazine for families and professionals. (Exceptional Parent, 65 East Route 9, River Edge, NJ 07661; tel: 201-489-4111; Internet: http://www.eparent.com/).

Parenting with a Disability. (Through the Looking Glass, 2198 Sixth Street, Suite 100, Berkeley, CA 94710; tel: 510-848-1112; 800-644-2666; Internet: www.lookingglass.org).

Agencies and Organizations

Consortium of Multiple Sclerosis Centers (CMSC) (c/o Gimbel MS Center at Holy Name Hospital, 718 Teaneck Road, Teaneck, NJ 07666; tel: 201-837-0727; Internet: www.mscare.org). The CMSC is made up of numerous MS centers throughout the United States and Canada. The Consortium's mission is to disseminate information to clinicians, increase resources and opportunities for research, and advance the standard of care for multiple sclerosis. The CMSC is a multidisciplinary organization, bringing together healthcare professionals from many fields involved in MS patient care.

Department of Veterans Affairs (VA) (810 Vermont Avenue, N.W., Washington, D.C. 20420; tel: 800-827-1000; Internet: www.va.gov). The VA provides a wide range of benefits and services to those who have served in the armed forces, their dependents, beneficiaries of deceased veterans, and dependent children of veterans with severe disabilities.

Equal Employment Opportunity Commission (EEOC) (Office of Communication and Legislative Affairs, 1801 L Street, N.W., 10th Floor, Washington, D.C. 20507; tel: 800-669-3362 [to order publications]; 800-669-4000 [to speak to an investigator]; 202-663-4900; Internet: www.eeoc.gov). The EEOC is responsible for monitoring the section of the ADA on employment regulations. Copies of the regulations are available.

Multiple Sclerosis Society of Canada (175 Bloor Street East, Suite 700, Toronto, Ontario M4W 3R8, Canada; tel: 416-922-6065; in Canada: 800-268-7582; Internet: www.mssociety.ca). A national organization that funds research, promotes public education, and produces publications in both English and French. They provide an "ASK MS Information System" database of articles on a wide variety of topics including treatment, research, and social services. Regional divisions and chapters are located throughout Canada.

Health Resource Center for Women with Disabilities (Rehabilitation Institute of Chicago, 345 East Superior Street, Chicago, IL 60611; tel: 312-908-7997; Internet: www.ric.org). The Center is a project run by and for women with disabilities. It publishes a free newsletter, "Resourceful Women," and offers support groups and educational seminars addressing issues from a disabled woman's perspective. Among its many educational resources, the Center has developed a video on mothering with a disability.

National Council on Disability (NCD) (1331 F Street, N.W., Suite 850, Washington, D.C. 20004; tel: 202-272-2004; Internet: www.ncd.gov). The Council is an independent federal agency whose role is to study and make recommendations about public policy for people with disabilities. Publishes a free newsletter, "Focus."

National Family Caregivers Association (NFCA) (10400 Connecticut Avenue, #500, Kensington, MD 20895; tel: 800-896-3650; Internet: www.thefamilycaregiver.org). NFCA is dedicated to improving the quality of life of America's 18,000,000 caregivers. It publishes a quarterly newsletter, a resource guide, and an information clearinghouse.

National Multiple Sclerosis Society (NMSS) (733 Third Avenue, New York, NY 10017; tel: 800-FIGHT MS; Internet: www.nmss.org). The NMSS is a nonprofit organization that supports national and international research into the prevention, cure, and treatment of MS. The Society's goals include provision of nationwide services to assist people with MS and their families, and provision of information to those with MS, their families, professionals, and the public. The programs and services of the Society promote knowledge, health, and independence while providing education and emotional support:

- ► Toll-free access to you by calling 800-FIGHT MS (800-344-4867).
- ► Internet Website with updated information about treatments, current research, and programs (http://www.nationalmssociety.org); local home page in many areas.
- ► Knowledge Is Power—An eight-segment, learn-at-home program (serial mailings) for people newly diagnosed with MS and their families.
- ► MS Learn Online—Online, interactive web casts on a wide variety of topics.
- ► Printed materials on a variety of topics available by calling 800-FIGHT-MS (800-344-4867) or in the library section of the National MS Society Website at http://www.nationalmssociety.org/library.asp.
- ► Educational programs on various topics throughout the year, provided through individual chapters.
- ► Annual national education conference, provided through individual chapters.
- ► Swimming and other exercise programs sponsored or co-

sponsored by some chapters, or referral to existing programs in the community.

► Wellness programs in some chapters.

National Park Service, U.S. Department of the Interior (P.O. Box 37127, Washington, D.C. 20013-7127; Internet: www.nps.gov). The service provides you with a listing of national parks and numbers for you to call to obtain up-to-date accessibility information for the individual parks.

Office on the Americans with Disabilities Act (Department of Justice, Civil Rights Division, P.O. Box 66118, Washington, D.C. 20035; tel: 202-514-0301; Internet: www.ada.gov). This office is responsible for enforcing the ADA.

Paralyzed Veterans of America (PVA) (801 Eighteenth Street N.W., Washington, D.C. 20006; tel: 800-424-8200; Internet: www.pva.org). PVA is a national information and advocacy agency working to restore function and quality of life for veterans with spinal cord dysfunction. It supports and funds education and research and has a national advocacy program that focuses on accessibility issues. PVA publishes brochures on many issues related to rehabilitation.

Social Security Administration (6401 Security Boulevard, Baltimore, MD 21235; tel: 800-772-1213; Internet: www.ssa.gov). To apply for social security benefits based on disability, call this office or visit your local social security branch office. The Office of Disability within the Social Security Administration publishes a free brochure entitled "Social Security Regulations: Rules for Determining Disability and Blindness."

Through the Looking Glass: National Research and Training Center on Families of Adults with Disabilities (2198 Sixth Street, Suite 100, Berkeley, CA 94710; tel: 510-848-4445; 800-644-2666; Internet: www.lookingglass.org).

United Spinal (formerly EPVA) (75-20 Astoria Boulevard, Jackson Heights, NY 11370; tel: 718-803-EPVA; Internet: www.unitedspinal. org). EPVA is a private, nonprofit organization dedicated to serving the needs of its members as well as other people with disabilities. While offering a wide range of benefits to member veterans with spinal cord dysfunction (including hospital liaison, sports and recreation, wheelchair repair, adaptive architectural consultations, research and educational services, communications, and library and information services, they will also provide brochures and information on a variety of subjects, free of charge to the general public.

Well Spouse Foundation (63 West Main St, Suite H, Freehold, NJ 07728; tel: 800-838-0879; Internet: www.wellspouse.org). An emotional support network for people married to or living with a chronically ill partner. Advocacy for home health and long-term care and a newsletter are among the services offered.

Assistive Technology

Access to Recreation: Adaptive Recreation Equipment for the Physically Challenged (2509 E. Thousand Oaks Boulevard, Suite 430, Thousand Oaks, CA 91362; tel: 800-634-4351; Internet: www.accesstr.com). Products include exercise equipment and assistive devices for sports, environmental access, games, crafts, and hobbies.

adaptABILITY (Department 2082, 75 Mill Street, Colchester, CT 06415; tel: 800-937-3482; Internet: www.adaptability.com). A free catalog of assistive devices and self-care equipment designed to enhance independence.

Adaptive Parenting: Idea Book I (Though the Looking Glass, 2198 Sixth Street, Suite 100, Berkeley, CA 94710; tel: 510-848-1112; 800-644-2666).

American Automobile Association (1712 G Street N.W., Washington, D.C. 20015; Internet: www.AAA.com). The AAA will provide a list of automobile hand-control manufacturers.

American Medical Alert (3265 Lawson Blvd., Oceanside, NY 11572; tel: 800-286-2622; Internet: www.amacalert.com). Personal emergency response system that links a person living alone with a 24-hour emergency response center, as well as other services.

Interim In-Touch (1601 Sawgrass Corporate Parkway, Sunrise, FL 33323; tel: 800-338-7786; Internet: www.interimhealthcare.com). Personal emergency response system that links a person living alone with a 24-hour emergency response center as well as other services.

Lifeline Systems, Inc. (111 Lawrence St., Framingham, MA 01702; tel: 508-988-1000; Internet: www.lifelinesys.com). Personal emergency response system that links a person living alone with a 24-hour emergency response center, as well as other services.

Life Enhancement Technologies, LLC, (807 Aldo Ave., Suite 101, Santa Clara, CA 95054; tel: 408-336-6940; Internet: www.2bcool.com). The company manufactures a variety of cooling suits that can be used in management of heat-related symptoms in MS.

Medic Alert Foundation International (2323 Colorado Ave., Turlock, CA 95382; tel: 888-633-4298; 209-668-3333; Internet: www.medicalert. org). A medical identification tag worn to identify a person's medical condition, medications, and any other important information that might be needed in case of an emergency. A file of the person's health data is maintained in a central database to be accessed by a physician or other emergency personnel who need to know the person's pertinent medical information.

National Rehabilitation Information Center (NARIC) (4200 Forbes Blvd., Suite 202, Lanham, MD 20706; tel: 800-346-2742 or 301-459-5900; Internet: www.naric.com).

NARIC is a library and information center on disability and rehabilitation, funded by the *National Institute on Disability and Rehabilitation Research* (NIDRR). NARIC operates two databases—ABLEDATA and REHABDATA. NARIC collects and disseminates the results of federally funded research projects and has a collection that includes commercially published books, journal articles, and audiovisual materials. NARIC is committed to serving both professionals and consumers who are interested in disability and rehabilitation. Information specialists can answer simple information requests and provide referrals immediately and at no cost. More complex database searches are available at nominal cost.

- ► ABLEDATA (8630 Fenton Street, Suite 930, Silver Spring, MD 20910; tel: 301-608-8992; 800-227-0216; fax: 301-608-8958; Internet: www.abledata.com). ABLEDATA is a national database of information on assistive technology designed to enable persons with disabilities to identify and locate the devices that will assist them in their home, work, and leisure activities. Information specialists are available to answer questions during regular business hours. ABLE INFORM BBS is available twenty-four hours a day to customers with a computer, modem, and telecommunications software.
- ► REHABDATA (8455 Colesville Road, Suite 935, Silver Spring, MD 20910; tel: 800-346-2742; Internet: www.naric.com/naric/search/rhab/browse.html). REHABDATA is a database containing bibliographic records with abstracts and summaries of the materials contained in the NARIC library of disability rehabilita-

tion materials. Information specialists are available to conduct a database search on any rehabilitation related topic.

RESNA: Rehabilitation, Engineering, and Assistive Technology Society of North America (1700 North Moore Street, Suite 1540, Arlington, VA 22209-1903; tel: 703-524-6686, P.O. Box 969, Etobicoke Station U, Etobicoke, Ontario M82 5P9; Internet: www.resna.org). RESNA is an international association for the advancement of rehabilitation technology. Their objectives are to improve the quality of life for the disabled through the application of science and technology and to influence policy relating to the delivery of technology to disabled persons. They will respond by mail to specific questions about modifying existing equipment and designing new devices.

SOS Wireless Communication (P.O. Box 15750, Irvine CA 92623; tel: 714-775-9400; Internet: www.sosphone.com). This mobile emergency response system operates on the existing national cellular network, providing 24-hour personalized service, nationwide roadside service, and free 911 calls.

Environmental Adaptations

A Consumer's Guide to Home Adaptation (Adaptive Environments Center, 374 Congress Street, Suite 301, Boston, MA 02210; tel: 617-695-1225; Internet: www.adaptenv.org). A workbook for planning adaptive home modifications such as lowering kitchen countertops and widening doorways.

American Institute of Architects (AIA) (1735 New York Avenue, N.W., Washington, D.C. 20006; tel: 800-242-3837; Internet: www.aia.org; e-mail: infocentral@aia.org). This organization will make referrals to architects who are familiar with the design requirements of people with disabilities.

Financing Home Accessibility Modifications (Center for Universal Design, North Carolina State University, Box 8613, Raleigh, NC 27695; tel: 919-515-3082; Internet: www.design.ncsu.edu/cud/). This publication identifies state and local sources of financial assistance for homeowners (or tenants) who need to make modifications in their homes.

GE Answer Center (9500 Williamsburg Plaza, Louisville, KY 40222; tel: 800-626-2000; Internet: www.geappliances.com). The Center, which is open twenty-four hours a day, seven days a week, offers assistance to individuals with disabilities as well as the general public. They offer two free brochures, "Appliance Help for Those with Special Needs," and "Basic Kitchen Planning for the Physically Handicapped."

National Association of Home Builders (NAHB) (NAHB Research Center, Economics and Policy Analysis Division, 1201 15th Street, NW Washington, DC 20005; tel: 800-368-5242; fax: 202-266-8559 Internet: www.nahb.com). The Research Center produces publications and provides training on housing and special needs. A publication entitled "Homes for a Lifetime" includes an accessibility checklist, financing options, and recommendations for working with builders and remodelers.

National Kitchen and Bath Association (687 Willow Grove Street, Hackettstown, NJ 07840; tel: 800-843-6522; Internet: www.nkba.org). The association produces a technical manual of barrier-free planning and has directories of certified designers and planners.

Travel

Accessible Journeys (tel: 800-846-4537 or 610-521-0339; Internet: www.disabilitytravel.com). A company that arranges travel for mobility-impaired travelers, and is affiliated with a network of offices in nine European countries.

Directory of Travel Agencies for the Disabled. (Written by Helen Hecker, published by Twin Peaks Press, P.O. Box 129, Vancouver, WA 98666-0129). This directory lists travel agents who specialize in arranging travel plans for people with disabilities.

The Disability Bookshop (P.O. Box 129, Vancouver, WA 98666; tel: 360-694-2462). The Disability Bookshop has an extensive list of books for disabled travelers, dealing with such topics as accessibility, travel agencies, accessible van rentals, medical resources, air travel, and guides to national parks.

Information for Handicapped Travelers (available free of charge from the National Library Service for the Blind and Physically Handicapped, 1291 Taylor Street, N.W., Washington, D.C. 20542; tel: 800-424-8567; 202-707-5100; Internet: www.loc.gov/nls/; e-mail: nls@loc.gov). A booklet providing information about travel agents, transportation, and information centers for individuals with disabilities.

Project Action (Internet: www.projectaction.org). Maintains a database on its website of information about the availability of accessible transportation anywhere in the United States. Users can highlight the state and city they plan to visit and view all transportation services available to them. The database also includes travel agencies specializing in travel arrangements for people with disabilities.

Society for the Advancement of Travel for the Handicapped (SATH) (347 Fifth Avenue, Suite 610, New York, NY 10016; tel: 212-447-7284; Internet: www.sath.org). SATH is a nonprofit organization that acts as a clearinghouse for accessible tourism information and is in contact with organizations in many countries to promote the development of facilities for disabled people. SATH publishes a quarterly magazine, "Access to Travel."

Travel for the Disabled: A Handbook of Travel Resources and 500 Worldwide Access Guides. (Written by Helen Hecker, published by Twin Peaks Press, P.O. Box 129, Vancouver, WA 98666; tel: 360-694-2462). The handbook provides information for disabled travelers about accessibility.

Travel Information Service (Moss Rehabilitation Hospital, 1200 West Tabor Road, Philadelphia, PA 19141; tel: 215-456-9900). The service provides information and referrals for people with disabilities.

Travelin' Talk (P.O. Box 1796 Wheat Ridge, CO 80034; tel: 303-232-2979; Internet: www.travelintalk.net). A network of more than one thousand people and organizations around the world who are willing to provide assistance to travelers with disabilities and share their knowledge about the areas in which they live. Travelin' Talk publishes a newsletter by the same name and has an extensive resource directory.

Wilderness Inquiry (808 14th Ave., S.E., Minneapolis, MN 55414; tel: 800-728-0719; 612-676-9400). Sponsors trips into the wilderness for people with disabilities or chronic conditions.

Visual Impairment

Canadian National Institute for the Blind (CNIB) (1929 Bayview Avenue, Toronto, Ontario M4G 3E8, Canada; tel: 416-486-2500; Internet: www.cnib.ca). The Institute provides counseling and rehabilitation services for Canadians with any degree of functional visual impairment. They offer public information literature and operate resource and technology centers. The national office has a list of provincial and local CNIB offices.

Lighthouse International (111 E. 59th Street, New York, NY 10022-1202; tel: 800-829-0500; TTY: 212-821-9713; Internet: www.lighthouse. org). Product catalog offers a wide variety of products for individuals with low vision.

The Library of Congress, Division for the Blind and Physically Handicapped (1291 Taylor Street, N.W., Washington, D.C. 20542; tel: 800-424-8567; 800-424-9100; for application: 202-287-5100; Internet: www.loc.gov/nls/). The library service provides free talking book equipment on loan as well as a full range of recorded books for individuals with disabilities or visual impairment. It also provides a variety of free library services through 140 cooperating libraries.

Publishing Companies Specializing in Health and Disability Issues

Demos Medical Publishing (386 Park Avenue South, Suite 201, New York, NY 10016; tel: 800-532-8663; Internet: www.demosmedpub.com).

Grey House Publishing (185 Millerton Road, P.O. Box 860, Millerton, NY 12546; tel: 800-562-2139; fax: 860-435-3004; e-mail: www.greyhouse.com).

Resources for Rehabilitation (22 Bonad Rd., Winchester, MA 01890; tel: 781-368-9094; Internet: www.rfr.org).

Twin Peaks Press (P.O. Box 129, Vancouver, WA 98666; tel: 360-694-2462; e-mail: TwinPeak@pacifier.com).

Woodbine House (Publishers of the Special-Needs Collection) (6510 Bells Mill Road, Bethesda, MD 20817; tel: 301-897-3570; 800-843-7323; Internet: www.woodbinehouse.com).

Professional Biographies of the Authors

Kathy Birk, M.D.

Kathy Birk attended Washington University in St. Louis, Missouri. She remained in Missouri for medical school where, during the first year, she experienced her first symptoms of multiple sclerosis (MS). She completed medical school in 1987 and moved onto her residency in obstetrics and gynecology in Rochester, New York. During her residency, Dr. Birk cared for two women with MS who were concerned that becoming pregnant might worsen their disease. Sharing their concern, Dr. Birk opted to begin the search for an answer about why pregnant women had fewer exacerbations than non-pregnant women, and about their long-term outcomes. Although her research did not identify any protective hormone or protein, she was able to demonstrate that having MS was not a sufficient reason for women to avoid becoming pregnant. Dr. Birk had her first child at the end of her residency.

Following residency, Dr. Birk practiced primary care office gynecology, delivered babies, and practiced surgery. Beginning in 1994, she had a series of mild relapses and that, along with significant fatigue, encouraged her to restrict her practice to the office setting. She subsequently retired from medical practice following a significant seizure that left her unable to be the active and involved physician she had always been. Within her first year of retirement, she was once again very busy—serving on boards of not-for-profit agencies, writing for the professional and lay literature, and presenting at conferences.

Dr. Birk's interest and involvement in MS grew out of her own personal experience as well as that of her grandmother, who lived most of her adult life with the disease. Dr. Birk has dedicated this chapter to her grandmother's memory.

Jack Burks, M.D

Jack Burks is a neurologist in Reno, Nevada who has specialized in multiple sclerosis (MS) for over 30 years. He was founder and President/CEO of one of the first comprehensive MS centers in the United States. His interest in neurology, rehabilitation, and chronic diseases underlies his work with families living with MS. Dr. Burks has lectured and written extensively in the field, including editing one of the latest textbooks on MS, *Multiple Sclerosis: Diagnosis, Medical Management, and Rehabilitation* (Demos Medical Publishing, 2000).

Dr. Burks is a Clinical Professor of Neurology at the UNSM, Vice President/Chief Medical Officer of Multiple Sclerosis Association of American, President of MS Alliance, member Medical Advisory Board of the National Multiple Sclerosis Society, and founding member of the Consortium of MS Centers, past President of the American Society of Neuroradiology, past member of the Board of the American Academy of Neurology. In addition, he is President of Burks and Associated Health Care Consulting Group.

Laura Cooper, Esq.

Laura Cooper graduated from the University of Washington Law School in 1968. She has been a practicing attorney for the past 17 years, two as counsel to the Chairman of the Interstate Commerce Commission in Washington, D.C., eight focusing on disability rights and consumer-based health law on behalf of the National Multiple Sclerosis Society, and the past three in private practice in Eugene, Oregon. She has also served the National MS Society as life planning and legal consultant, special consultant on employment initiatives, and a member of the Services Subcommittee on Independent Living.

Ms. Cooper was teaching science on an Indian reservation when she first experienced gait problems, vertigo, numbness, and tingling. The severity of her MS forced her to leave her job at age 22. She enrolled in a couple of graduate school courses, paid her tuition with savings, and received support from the Department of Vocational Rehabilitation for wheelchair assistance. Her failing health put her in and out of hospitals and eventually, at age 23, into a nursing home. Three months later, Ms. Cooper found an ad in a newspaper for a wheelchair-accessible apartment complex. She negotiated for space, some furniture, a hospital bed, and a commode, which she ordered on an old Visa card, and used her Social Security payment to help pay the rent. Her parents helped her by purchasing a lift-equipped van.

Ms. Cooper applied to law school and received a full tuition scholarship to Gonzaga University in Spokane, Washington. While in law school, she experienced several exacerbations that left her temporarily blind and quadriplegic. She transferred to the University of Washington to finish her degree, following which she was named one of the twenty outstanding young American lawyers "who make a difference" by the American Bar Association. During her search for employment, Ms. Cooper received more than 400 rejections, until one law firm was willing to look at her abilities instead of her disabilities.

Peggy Crawford, Ph.D.

After completing her master's degree in Pediatric Nursing at Case Western Reserve University in 1976, Peggy Crawford worked for nearly a decade at Rainbow Babies and Children's Hospital as a pediatric nurse clinician in the area of diabetes and endocrinology. It was during this time that she developed her longstanding interest in how individuals and families cope with the day-to-day demands and challenges of chronic illness. After completing a PhD in Clinical Psychology at Kent State University and an internship in Health Psychology, Dr. Crawford completed a year of postdoctoral training in Health Psychology at the Mellen Center for MS Treatment and Research at the Cleveland Clinic Foundation in Cleveland, Ohio. For the next year, she was a faculty member in the Department of Family Medicine at Case Western Reserve University where her responsibilities included training family practice physicians in the behavioral science component of patient care.

Since 1993, Dr. Crawford has been a member of the professional staff at the Mellen Center where she is responsible for health psychology services including assessment and treatment (individual and group therapy) of individuals referred for a variety of concerns including emotional distress, stress-related symptoms, coping difficulties, and fatigue. She has conducted research on depression in patients taking beta interferon, group psychotherapy as a treatment modality in chronic illness, and psychosocial outcomes in MS and epilepsy surgery patients. Her publications have focused on issues related to coping with chronic illness and the psychological aspects of MS including depression and the special challenges involved in parenting with MS. Her ongoing interests include the identification of factors that contribute to effective coping with chronic illness, the impact of depression, and issues unique to women with chronic illness.

Frederick Foley, Ph.D.

Frederick Foley received his PhD in Clinical Psychology from Fordham University in 1986. Since then, he has been on the faculty at Albert Einstein College of Medicine and Ferkauf Graduate School of Psychology, both at Yeshiva University, in Bronx, NY. He is currently an associate professor of psychology.

Dr. Foley is the Director of Neuropsychology and Psychosocial Research at the Bernard Gimbel Comprehensive MS Center at Holy Name Hospital in Teaneck, NJ. Dr. Foley has dedicated his career to improving psychosocial rehabilitation and treatment methods in MS. His research projects have focused broadly on developing outcome measures and/or psychosocial treatments for depression, cognitive function, and sexual function in MS. The federal government and private foundations in the United States and England have funded his research.

Dr. Foley is on the board of directors of the Consortium of Multiple Sclerosis Centers, an international organization of MS professionals, and serves as Past-President for this organization. He has numerous publications and book chapters on his work in MS, and he has received recognition from the Academy of Psychosomatic Medicine for his research.

Barbara Giesser, M.D.

Barbara Giesser is an associate clinical professor of neurology at the UCLA School of Medicine. She received her bachelor's degree from the University of Miami, a master's degree from the University of Texas at Houston, and her medical degree from the University of Texas Medical School at San Antonio. She has specialized in the care of persons with MS since 1982, and trained at the MS Research and Training Center of the Albert Einstein College of Medicine, under the direction of Dr. Labe Scheinberg.

Dr. Giesser has served as Medical Director of the Gimbel MS Center at Holy Name Hospital in Teaneck, New Jersey, and Medical Director of the Rehab Institute of Tucson. She is currently an associate professor of clinical neurology at the University of California at Los Angeles and Medical Director of the Marilyn Hilton MS Achievement Center at UCLA. She has published in the areas of cognition in MS, bladder management and women's issues.

In addition to her clinical activities, Dr. Giesser has been active in developing educational materials about MS for medical student and residents, as well as in client and professional education endeavors for the National MS Society.

Deborah Hertz, M.P.H

Deborah Hertz has been the National Multiple Sclerosis Society's National Director of Medical Programs since October 1995, working to strengthen relationships with the medical community. In this role, she assists with development of Clinical Advisory Committees, works with MS clinics and centers throughout the United States, and supports the development of physical health and wellness programs. Ms. Hertz is currently on the editorial board for Real Living with MS and served a term on the editorial board for the MS Exchange, a newsletter for nurses. She has co-authored and authored chapters in two books on community resources for people with MS. She is also responsible for development of training materials for aquatics instructors interested in specialized programs for people with MS and is currently working on training materials for yoga instructors.

Ms. Hertz came to the National Multiple Sclerosis Society in

September 1994 to be the Director of the AmeriCorps program "Bridge to Independence." She came with extensive experience in developing and implementing community based health-care programs as well as in financial management of grants and contracts. Ms. Hertz received an undergraduate degree from Vassar College and a Master of Public Health degree (MPH) (with a major in long-term care administration) from Columbia University.

Nancy Holland, R.N., Ed.D.

Nancy Holland is vice president of the Clinical Programs Department at the National Multiple Sclerosis Society in New York. She earned a doctorate in higher and adult education from Teachers College, Columbia University, and holds undergraduate and graduate degrees in nursing. Dr. Holland received a Career Development Award from the National Institute on Disability and Rehabilitation Research and is author/editor of more than 60 MS-related articles, books and chapters including *Multiple Sclerosis: A Guide for Patients and Their Families*, *Multiple Sclerosis: A Guide for the Newly Diagnosed*, *Comprehensive Nursing Care in Multiple Sclerosis*, *Multiple Sclerosis: A Self-Care Guide to Wellness*, and *Multiple Sclerosis in Clinical Practice*. She is a founding member of the Board of Directors of the International Organization of MS Nurses (IOMSN), and chair of the IOMSN Research Committee.

Rosalind C. Kalb, Ph.D.

Rosalind Kalb, a clinical psychologist, is Director of the Professional Resource Center at the National Multiple Sclerosis Society in New York, developing and providing educational and consultation services to clinicians who care for people with MS. In her private clinical practice, she specializes in the needs of individuals and families living with chronic illness and disability.

After receiving her doctorate from Fordham University in New York City, she began her career in MS, providing individual, group, and family therapy at the MS Care Center at the Albert Einstein College of Medicine. Following the Center's relocation to New York Medical College, Dr. Kalb added a variety of other clinical and research activities to her work in MS, including groups for well spouses and couples living with MS, and neuropsychological evaluation and cognitive rehabilitation for research and treatment purposes. While at the Center, with funding from the National MS Society, Dr. Kalb investigated "The Impact of Multiple Sclerosis in Childhood and Adolescence." The study evaluated the effects of early-onset MS on intellectual function and academic performance, as well as a variety of psychosocial variables. Dr. Kalb also collaborated with Drs. Nicholas LaRocca and Charles Smith on a study, funded by the National Institute on Disability and Rehabilitation Research, entitled "The Psychosocial Impact of Parental Multiple Sclerosis on Children and Adolescents."

Dr. Kalb has authored or edited a number of publications about multiple sclerosis. She is the author of *Families Affected by Multiple Sclerosis: Disease Impacts and Coping Strategies*, a monograph published in 1995 by the National MS Society, and edits the Society's *Knowledge is Power* learn-at-home series for individuals newly diagnosed with MS. Dr. Kalb has edited two books—*Multiple Sclerosis: A Guide for Families*, published in 1998, and *Multiple Sclerosis: The Questions You Have, The Answers You Need*, initially published in 1996 and now in its third edition. She serves on the editorial board of several publications, including *Keep S'myelin*, the National MS Society newsletter for young children who have a parent with MS.

Kimberly Koch, M.P.A

Kimberly Koch, MPA is the Manager, Knowledge and Family Programs in the Client Programs Department of the National Multiple Sclerosis Society. She received her undergraduate degree in political science and international relations at the University of Wisconsin-Madison, and her Master of Public Administration in program planning and implementation at George Mason University.

Ms. Koch has over 18 years of professional experience, with over 14 years spent in program planning and implementation. Her areas of interest include programs for children and families, and she has developed and facilitated group programs for children and teenagers, and for adults who have parenting concerns. She has also been involved in welfare reform and child abuse prevention initiatives, and domestic violence prevention and awareness efforts.

Ms. Koch has been active with a variety of child and family welfare serving agencies, organizations, task forces, and commissions, both as program staff and various volunteer capacities. She has presented at local, state, and national conferences on child abuse prevention strategies.

Lauren Krupp, M.D.

Lauren Krupp is a professor of neurology at the State University of New York at Stony Brook. She is director of the National Pediatric Multiple Sclerosis Center at the Stony Brook University Hospital and co-director of the adult MS Center. She has been involved in the care of individuals with MS for over 20 years. After receiving her medical degree and neurology training from the Albert Einstein College of Medicine, Dr. Krupp completed a neuroimmunology and MS fellowship at the National Institutes of Health (NIH).

As a member of the medical school faculty at Stony Brook University, Dr. Krupp sees patients, teaches, and pursues clinical research. She has received research support from NIH, the National MS Society, and other funding agencies for studies on the nature and treatment of MS-related cognitive impairment, fatigue, and pediatric MS. Her interest in pediatric MS recently led to the establishment of the first multidisciplinary pediatric MS center in the United States. Dr. Krupp has numerous publications in the field of MS and is a frequent speaker at national and international scientific conferences.

Nicholas G. LaRocca, Ph.D.

Nicholas LaRocca, who received his doctorate in clinical psychology from Fordham University, has been the Director of Health Care Delivery and Policy Research at the National Multiple Sclerosis Society in New York City since 1997. Before coming to work for the National MS Society, he was Director of Research at the Research and Training Center for MS at St. Agnes Hospital, White Plains, New York and Associate Professor of Neurology and Medicine at New York Medical College.

Dr. LaRocca has extensive experience in both psychosocial research and psychological treatment in multiple sclerosis (MS). He has designed, administered, and analyzed a number of clinical studies in MS, including neurogenic bladder dysfunction, comparisons of inpatient and outpatient rehabilitation, and the role of stressful life events in MS. Dr.

LaRocca was principal investigator of a project funded by the National Institute on Disability and Rehabilitation Research entitled "The Comprehensive Rehabilitation of Cognitive Dysfunction in Multiple Sclerosis." He also served as principal investigator of a National MS Society-funded "Program to Facilitate Retention of Employment Among Persons with Multiple Sclerosis," and as co-principal investigator for the National MS Society-funded projects entitled "Development of a Multiple Sclerosis Quality of Life Measurement."

During his 25 years of work in MS, Dr. LaRocca has led support groups for persons with MS and their spouses and given innumerable workshops and presentations for both lay and professional audiences. In 1992, he was the invited speaker for the National MS Society audioteleconference entitled "Multiple Sclerosis: Understanding Your Mind and Emotions." He is the author of a number of scientific papers and book chapters and serves on the editorial boards of The Journal of Rehabilitation Research and Development, and Real Living with MS.

Deborah M. Miller, Ph.D., L.I.S.W.

Deborah M. Miller is Director of Comprehensive Care at the Mellen Center for MS Treatment and Research of the Cleveland Clinic. In this capacity, her responsibilities include program development and outcomes research, providing clinical care, conducting psychosocial research, and assuring integration of the Center's clinical, research, and operational activities. Dr. Miller obtained her MSSA and Ph.D. from the School of Applied Social Sciences, Case Western Reserve University.

A social worker with more than 20 years experience in the area of chronic disability, Dr. Miller has been a member of the Mellen Center's interdisciplinary care team since 1985. Her practice interests focus on marital and family adjustment to the consequences of MS. Her research interests include quality of life assessment, the impact of clinical interventions on health status, and the predictors of service utilization. She is currently the principal investigator for a NIH-funded study entitled "Using the Internet to Improve Patients' Self-Management of Chronic Illness."

Using her clinical experience, Dr. Miller has developed and facilitated group treatment programs for school age children and teenagers whose parents have MS, and for adults who have parenting concerns because of MS. She has lectured nationally on these subjects.

Dr. Miller has extensive affiliations with the National Multiple Sclerosis Society. She is a member of the Northeast Ohio Chapter's Client Services Committee and won that Chapter's "Health Care Professional" award in 1991. In addition, Dr. Miller is a past president and a current member of the Board of Trustees of the Long Term Care Ombudsman Program.

Elizabeth Morrison, M.D., M.S.Ed.

Elizabeth Morrison graduated from the Brown University School of Medicine in 1992. After medical school, she spent a year serving as the national president of the American Medical Student Association. Dr. Morrison completed her family medicine residency training in 1996 at Ventura County Medical Center and her Master's degree in medical education in 1998 at the University of Southern California-Keck School of Medicine. In 2001, the California Academy of Family Physicians named her Family Physician of the Year.

That same year, while Dr. Morrison was teaching at the University of California, Irvine, she was diagnosed with multiple sclerosis (MS). Through the National Multiple Sclerosis Society's Southern California Chapter, she started a support group for health professionals with MS and has given presentations on health maintenance in MS. Dr. Morrison is now completing a fellowship at the UCI Multiple Sclerosis Treatment Center and plans afterward to focus her clinical practice on MS care. She conducts research on exercise in MS, exploring the optimal exercise "dose" that is beneficial and safe for people with MS. In her spare time, she tries to practice what she preaches by cycling and hiking as often as possible.

Dorothy Northrop, M.S.W

Dorothy Northrop is Director of Clinical Programs for the National Multiple Sclerosis Society, coordinating Society initiatives to expand quality long-term care options and health insurance coverage for people with multiple sclerosis (MS). Prior to joining the home office, Ms. Northrop was Director of Chapter Services for the Greater North Jersey

Chapter of the Society for over five years, where she was responsible for implementing a comprehensive plan of services and programs for 4500 people with MS and their families.

Ms. Northrop received her B.A. in Sociology from the University of Massachusetts and her Masters Degree in Social Work from Columbia University in New York City. A licensed social worker in the state of New Jersey, she has served on the Multiple Sclerosis Advisory Council of Merck-Medco Managed Care, the Advisory Board of the Office of Disability Services in Bergen County, NJ, and as a consultant to community healthcare agencies and skilled nursing facilities. Ms. Northrop authored an article entitled "Managed Health Care: How Do Changes in the Health Care System Affect Patients with Multiple Sclerosis" in the Summer, 2001 issue of the Multiple Sclerosis Quarterly Report, and is co-author of the book "Health Insurance Resources: Options for People with a Chronic Disease or Disability" published by Demos Medical Publishing Inc. in 2003.

Faith Seidman, C.S.W

Faith Seidman has had MS for 19 years. As the divorced mother of two sons, and the daughter of two loving and supportive parents, she is acutely aware of the impact of the disease on the entire family.

After being out of school for 20 years, Ms. Seidman received her master's degree in social work from Adelphi University in 1997 (riding in her motorized scooter to claim her diploma).

INDEX

Note: Italic f indicates illustrations.

F

R

Resources, 6-9, 225-234, 245-258

S

V

Vardenafil (Levitra), 64
Vaseline, 57
Venlafaxine (Effexor), 20
Viagra. *See* sildenafil
Visual impairment, 257-258
Visual-spatial abilities, 26

W

We Magazine, 243
We're Accessible, 243
Weakness, sexuality and intimacy issues in, 73
Web sites of interest, 246-249
Weekly health promoting behaviors, 182, 183f
Weight control, 185-187
Wellbutrin. *See* bupropion
Well-Partner/Spouse Association, 160, 233, 253
Well-being. *See* general health and well-being, 181
Wilderness Inquiry, 257
Wills, 221-223
Word-finding problems, 25-26
Worst-case scenario planning, 198, 205-207

Y

Young Persons with MS, A Network for Families, 111-112, 228

Z

Zanaflex. tizanidine, 73
Zoloft. *See* sertraline